RESEARCH MONOGRAPHS ON HUMAN POPULATION BIOLOGY

General Editor: G. A. HARRISON

RESEARCH MONOGRAPHS ON HUMAN POPULATION BIOLOGY

THE STRUCTURE OF AN AFRICAN PASTORALIST COMMUNITY

Demography, History, and Ecology of the Ngamiland Herero

RENEE PENNINGTON

College of William and Mary, Williamsburg

and

HENRY HARPENDING

Pennsylvania State University

CLARENDON PRESS · OXFORD

1993

Oxford University Press, Walton Street, Oxford OX2 6DP
Oxford   New York   Toronto
Delhi   Bombay   Calcutta   Madras   Karachi
Kuala Lumpur   Singapore   Hong Kong   Tokyo
Nairobi   Dar es Salaam   Cape Town
Melbourne   Auckland   Madrid
and associated companies in
Berlin   Ibadan

Oxford is a trade mark of Oxford University Press

Published in the United States
by Oxford Univeresity Press Inc., New York

A catalogue record for this book is available from the British Library

Library of Congress Cataloging in Publication Data
Pennington, Renee.
The structure of an African pastoralist community: demography,
history, and ecology of the Ngamiland Herero / Renee Pennington,
Henry Harpending.
(Research monographs on human population biology)
Includes bibliographical references and index.
1. Herero (African people)–Population. 2. Fertility, Human–
Botswana. I. Harpending, Henry. II. Title. III. Series.
DT2458.H47P46   1993   304.6'08996399–dc20   93-15644

ISBN 0-19-852286-X (cloth)

Typeset by the authors using L^AT_EX
Printed in Great Britain by Biddles Ltd, Guildford & King's Lynn

Preface

The production of this manuscript was financially supported in two phases. Pennington's field-work among the Herero of Botswana in 1987–9 was supported by grants for dissertation research from the Wenner-Gren Foundation for Anthropological Research and the Hill Fund of the Pennsylvania State University. Both of us received support from a grant from the National Institutes on Aging (AG03110) to Jennie Keith and Christine Fry. Pennington received support during the writing phase from the National Institute of Child Health and Human Development through a grant for core support of population research (HD-05876) and a training grant (HD-07014) to the Center for Demography and Ecology, University of Wisconsin.

Many individuals helped during various stages of our research. We are especially grateful to the Office of the President in Gaborone for permission to carry out our field-work and to Tjako Mpulubusi and others at the National Museum and Art Gallery for support and encouragement. We are indebted to the Herero and Mbanderu for their co-operation and interest in our project. The Lutheran Medical Clinic in Sehitwa provided invaluable assistance during our field-work by providing housing and logistic support.

We thank the many other individuals who provided us with comments, technical assistance and logistic support. Robert Aunger, Robert Bailey, Stephen Beckerman, Gillian Bentley, Nicholas Blurton Jones, Anne Buchanan, Elizabeth Cashdan, Clifford Clogg, Douglas Crewes, Patricia Draper, Rada Dyson-Hudson, Elliot Fratkin, Timothy Gage, Kristen Hawkes, Kim Hill, Christine Himes, Holly Hughes, Nancy Howell, Pierre Jamagne, Reginah Kaevarua, Susan Kent, George Kephart, Enamuuharari Korujezu, Timon Korujezu, Uakapita Korujezu, Barthelemy Kuate Defo, Xashe Kumsa, Jeffrey Kurland, Xuma Kxau, Richard Lee, Bruce Lindsay, Manuel Marenga, Katjambungu Mbatara, Antonio McDaniel, Phillemon Motsu, Arindam Mukherjee, Kaetiramukuao Ndjarakana, Gakekgosi Otugile, Alberto Palloni, Elliot Posner, David Reed, Kenneth Rizzi, Alan Rogers, Ida Simon, Himla Soodyall, Mark Stoneking, Kukaora Tjeja, Samuel Tjeja, Titus Tjirongo, David Tracer, Mitchell Tropila, James Vaupel, Linda Vigilant, Deborah Walker, Kenneth Weiss, and James Wood especially provided assistance. Most of all, we gratefully acknowledge the help we have had from our families.

Several chapters of this monograph draw heavily on individual articles we published in journals. Parts of Chapter 2, where our field methods are described, and much of the chapter on infant and child mortality (Chapter 3) originally appeared in *Human Biology* in 1991.[1] Chapters 5 and 6 on Herero fertility were drawn from a single manuscript that we published in 1991 in the *American Journal of Human Biology*.[2] In Chapter 8 we describe Herero child fosterage practices from an evolutionary perspective. This chapter was based on a 1991 *Ethology and Sociobiology* manuscript.[3] Chapter 9 compares the demography of the Herero with their !Kung neighbors and explores the viability of the !Kung ecological models in light of our Herero findings. Much of this chapter is taken from a 1992 *Human Biology* paper.[4] Chapter 10 is written around a 1991 *Social Biology* paper.[5] This final chapter pulls together the demographic data from the preceeding chapters. In re-using the previously published material, we have tried to integrate rather than re-hash our earlier work. While striving for continuity throughout the monograph, we hope that each chapter is relatively self-contained and separately readable.

Williamsburg   R.P.
State College   H.H.
May 1993

---

[1] Reprinted in part by permission of the publisher from 'Age structure and sex-biased mortality among Herero pastoralists', by H. Harpending and R. Pennington, *Human Biology* **63**, 329–53. Copyright 1991 by Wayne State University Press.

[2] Reprinted in part by permission of the publisher from 'Infertility in Herero pastoralists of Southern Africa', by R. Pennington and H. Harpending, *American Journal of Human Biology* **3**, 135–53. Copyright 1991 by Wiley-Liss, Inc.

[3] Reprinted in part by permission of the publisher from 'Child fostering as a reproductive strategy among southern African pastoralists', by R. Pennington, *Ethology and Sociobiology* **12**, 83–104. Copyright 1991 by Elsevier Science Publishing Co., Inc.

[4] Reprinted in part by permission of the publisher from 'Did food increase fertility? An evaluation of !Kung and Herero history', by R. Pennington, *Human Biology* **64**, 497–521. Copyright 1991 by Wayne State University Press.

[5] Reprinted in part by permission of the publisher from 'Effect of infertility on the population structure of the Herero and Mbanderu of Southern Africa', by R. Pennington and H. Harpending, *Social Biology* **38**, 127–39.

Contents

Figures

Tables

1
Introduction and background

Introduction

This monograph is about the ecology and population dynamics of a group of cattle and goat herders in the northern Kalahari Desert of the Ngamiland District of Botswana (see Fig. 1.1). Although the Herero[1] arrived in this region less than a century ago as destitute refugees, these staunchly traditional Bantu speakers have established themselves as a prominent and prosperous tribe in a pocket of the Kalahari previously occupied almost exclusively by !Kung-speaking foragers. Their rise to economic prominence in Botswana has been accompanied by dramatic decreases in mortality and increases in fertility, and a resurgence of tribal ethnicity.

Our demographic data were collected through intense ethnographic interviews of over 700 Herero living in north-western Botswana. Studies such as ours illustrate the trade-offs between large-scale censuses that traditional demographers are comfortable with and small qualitative studies familiar to anthropologists and sociologists. Statistics from large national or regional studies that blur distinctions among genetically, historically, and economically different groups may not reveal much about the processes that generated them because differences *within* groups are confounded by differences *between* groups. For example, Herero mortality rates are low by the national standards of Botswana, yet those of their neighbours the !Kung Bushmen[2] are relatively high. Neither the difference between the ethnic groups nor their causes, which we describe in Chapters 4 and 9, is apparent from census data alone. Our methods and the use of traditional Herero year names allowed us to date with confidence the years of birth of our informants and the years of vital events of their family members in a part of the world where this information is generally unknown.

In turn, demographic data provide information about culture that is missed by ethnography. In Chapter 3 we describe drastic differences in

---

[1] We use the term 'Herero' to refer to the two closely-related tribes of Herero speakers in Botswana, the Herero and Mbanderu. The important differences between these two groups of pastoralists are discussed later in this chapter.

[2] Recent literature in anthropology substitutes *San* for Bushmen. We do not follow this practice because San is a very impolite form of reference in the Kalahari. Bushmen are also known by their Tswana name, *Basarwa* or *Sarwa*, in the literature. Herero call them *Ovakuruha*.

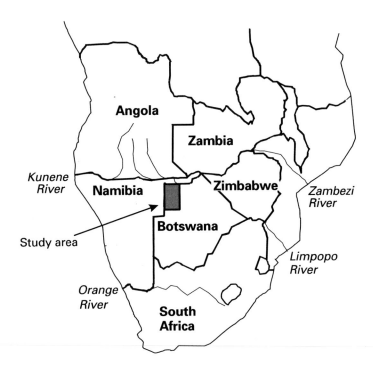

Fig. 1.1. Location of western Ngamiland in Africa.

the survival of infants in favour of females. Although the sex differential suggests a preference for females in Herero society, people neither admit offspring sex preferences nor overtly prefer one sex over the other. Similarly, the relationships among historically low Herero fertility, marital instability, and high rates of non-marital child-bearing are vital to our understanding of child fosterage, marriage, kinship, and inheritance in Herero society.

Most important, demographic rates determine the age and sex structure of the social environment of individuals and how their environment changes over the life-span. We cannot understand maternal and paternal behaviours, for example, without knowledge of the probability faced by parents that an infant will still be alive six months or six years in the future. This traditional role of demography in the social sciences has recently been supplemented and, to an extent, supplanted in anthropology by a focus on individual strategizing and the biological roots of social institutions. Human evolutionary ecology has directed attention to understanding the Darwinian fitness of individuals and its correlates. Fitness is measured from rates of birth and death, so good human ecology must start with demography.

We recognize that societies are not organic wholes but are collections of individuals who have sometimes competing and sometimes identical interests. The old functionalist notion that societies are like organisms and that individuals work together as if they were cells in an organism is flawed because cells in an organism share the same genetic material (Dawkins 1976) and have identical reproductive interests. Individual mammals, at the most fundamental level of genetic code, share overlapping but not identical genetic material so that unconstrained co-operation could not evolve.

Cultural transmission of values and goals transforms this underlying conflict between genetic individuality and social cohesion. It is not so clear, however, how far it is transformed. Is social life to be understood as reproductive competition overlaid with a veneer of sociality? On the other hand is human social ability and interaction so contingent on the corpus of learned material that the Darwinian motives are buried, suppressed, and irrelevant? We are fairly agnostic about this issue, but such questions motivate our demographic interests. The Darwinian metric of success is the fitness of individuals, and demography is really the study of fitness and the covariates of fitness.

Most of our informants were very interested in our study and in the issues that we were studying. They were not so agnostic about the relative importance of social and biological determinants of behaviour, but the two sexes had rather different perspectives. Many Herero women are directly concerned with fitness, with genetic relationship, and with reproductive success. Many men, on the other hand, are much more interested in social wealth and power. It was striking to us that so much of the cultural anthropology of Africa that we had read before beginning the study was like the perceptions and statements of Herero men but not of Herero women, as if the bulk of it had been generated by talking with the male half of society. There is more discussion of these issues in Chapter 7.

Our aims are thus descriptive, methodological, and theoretical. In the following chapters, we develop non-traditional methods for extracting information from a single body of demographic data and use the estimates of vital rates to infer trends in the life history of people in the region. We frequently employ an evolutionary perspective in our interpretations, and we provide ethnographic and historical context.

In the next section we provide an overview of our field-work. The remainder of the chapter traces the origins of the Herero from the beginnings of the Bantu expansion into Southern Africa to the present. We use linguistic, archaeological, historical, and biological evidence to identify the role of Herero in Southern African history and prehistory. Although the Herero are just one of many peoples in Africa, our study provides an additional data point in the sketchy African historical picture. The last section of this chapter is an overview of Herero culture.

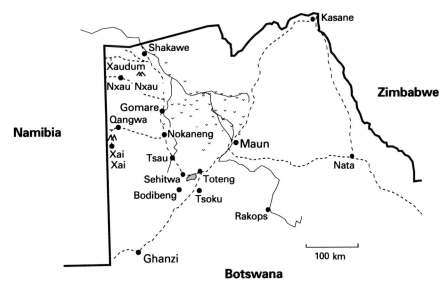

Fig. 1.2.   Major villages and named settlements in western Ngamiland in this study.

Field-work

The Herero pastoralists in Botswana are actually divided into two tribal groups, the Herero and the Mbanderu. Although many of them prefer the distinction, we regard them as a single ethnic group because we were unable to detect any strong differences in language or customs between them. We will refer to members of the Herero tribe as Herero *proper* when we wish to distinguish them from the other groups of Herero speakers in Botswana, Namibia, and Angola.

The Herero in this study live in the areas of Ngamiland west of the Okavango Delta indicated on the map in Fig. 1.2. The Herero are a minority group in Ngamiland and Botswana, albeit a prominent one. Along the delta and throughout the desert they interact with Tawana (northern Tswana), Yei, Mbukushu, and other Bantu-speaking groups. There are also large settlements of Khoisan-speaking peoples, especially !Kung Bushmen well known to anthropologists, in the western and northern parts of our study area.

Our project began when Harpending was recruited as a collaborator in a multicultural study of ageing. The goal of the study, organized by Christine Fry and Jennie Keith, was to understand the relations among age groups and the meaning of age categories in different parts of the world (Ikels *et al.* 1987; Keith *et al.* 1988). One of our most interesting findings that reflects on the issue of ageing (see Chapter 4) is the extraordinary vigour and durability of Herero elderly. The longevity of the elderly is a biological indicator of the respect, honour, and good care that old people receive in this society and is an important constraint on the lives of children and younger people.

Harpending's field-work began in July 1987 and continued through August 1988. Pennington arrived in March 1988 to do a 12-month demographic and ethnographic study of fertility, child fosterage, and marriage. While Harpending maintained a base camp in the Qangwa valley in the extreme west of Ngamiland, Pennington lived at the Lutheran mission station in Sehitwa at the southern perimeter of the Okavango. Since our population was dispersed over approximately 60 000 km^2, we did most of our actual interviewing on the road, living in tents or staying in huts that were temporarily empty and available. A vehicle with four-wheel drive was necessary to traverse occasional deep sand year-round and treacherous mud during the rainy season.

We standardized the basic parts of our questionnaires early in our field-work, and we maintained separate databases on portable microcomputers in the same format. Periodically we cross-checked overlapping information for consistency and replicability. Altogether we interviewed over 700 men and women in Ngamiland and ascertained 3500 Herero living in the region. There are 10 000–15 000 Herero in the whole of Botswana (see Chapter 10), most of whom live in Ngamiland.

Herero origins

The Herero are part of one of the great population expansions in history, the movement of Bantu-speaking people from West Africa into central, eastern, and Southern Africa. To understand Herero demography today it is necessary to discuss aspects of the prehistory and history of this event. The Herero are part of the south-western Bantu group, related to people in northern Namibia, Angola, Zambia, and the Okavango region of Botswana. Genetic evidence and regional history suggest that they have been a small group isolated from their neighbours for a very long time. We will suggest later that pathological sterility in the region may account for these and other aspects of Herero history and population dynamics.

The circumstances of the migration of Herero from South West Africa (now Namibia) to the Bechuanaland Protectorate (now Botswana) at the turn of the century will prove to be important to our understanding of the present-day population structure. The signature of the age pattern of wartime mortality persists, and we will infer the demographic and historical significance of the movement of Herero into Bechuanaland from our estimates of vital rates derived throughout the monograph. We will also

suggest that our demographic data and the depth of the historical roots of
this group in the region contradict the widely held belief that Africa has
been characterized by very high fertility and mortality in past centuries.

The migration to Botswana

Before the Herero–German War of 1904–07 very few Herero lived outside
South West Africa and southern Angola, although they occasionally grazed
livestock in other territories. The Herero apparently possessed large herds
of cattle in South West Africa that were the source of ongoing disputes
among factions of Herero and other tribal groups (Vedder 1966*b*; Sundermeier 1986). The German colonial effort late in the nineteenth century,
however, impinged too deeply on their autonomy, leading to the Herero
revolt in January of 1904.

Following the critical defeat of the Herero in the Battle of Waterberg
(see the map in Fig. 1.3) in August of 1904, they dispersed, many of them
trekking north and east across the waterless region to Bechuanaland. Although many died of thirst or starvation during the flight, tens of thousands
of those remaining in South West Africa became the victims of German patrols under orders to seek out and kill all Herero. Sources estimate that
there were 70 000–85 000 Herero in South West Africa before the war (Bley
1971; Bridgeman 1981; Drechsler 1980) and only 15 000–25 000 at its conclusion (Bridgeman 1981; Drechsler 1980). The number of Herero who
escaped to what is now Botswana is unknown, but the number of refugees
is upward of 1800, and there may have been as many as 9000 (Chapter 10).

The major influx of Herero occurred in 1904–05 following the defeat
at Waterberg. Samuel Maharero, a prominent leader among the Herero
proper, led a group of followers to Bechuanaland by way of the Eiseb River
(Sundermeier 1986). Several groups of Herero are known to have passed
through Qangwa throughout the next year (Howell 1979; Lee 1979). None
of them stayed, choosing to move on to Tsau and the Lake Ngami area
instead. Lee (1979) learned of one group of Herero who were chased as
far east as Gura and Gautsha in Nyae Nyae by the German patrols. The
patrols turned back thinking they had reached British territory when they
encountered Tswana cattleposts. Another large group apparently followed
Nicodemus Nguvauva, a leader among the Mbanderu (Sundermeier 1986).

Larger numbers of Herero left South West Africa by way of Rietfontein,
hoping to settle in Ghanzi. The British did not allow the Herero to stay
because Ghanzi had already been set aside for Boers (Tlou 1985). Instead,
the Tawana Chief Sekgoma allowed them to settle in Sehitwa and Nokaneng. Sekgoma, the leader of the Tswana tribe in political control of what is
now essentially Ngamiland, allowed the Herero to have their own headman,
who was ultimately responsible to Sekgoma. Several Herero told us that
they came to Tawana territory because of historical agreements between

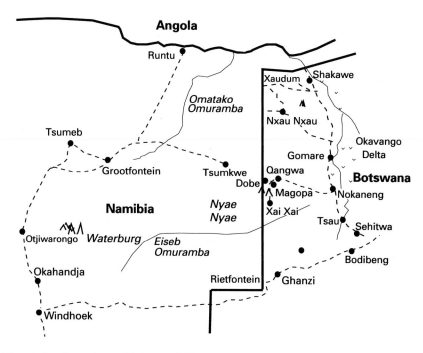

Fig. 1.3. Locations of historical Herero migrations.

Herero and Tawana leaders in which each group was to be given refuge in the other's territory. These agreements are also described in Tlou (1985) and Sundermeier (1986).

Most of the Herero initially settled near Lake Ngami. Today, the Herero proper are concentrated near Makakung while Mbanderu tend to live near Sehitwa. Many families have since expanded into the more remote Xai Xai, Qangwa, Nxau Nxau, and Xaudum valleys in western and north-western Ngamiland. Most people migrated after 1950, probably initiated by tsetse fly outbreaks along the Okavango Delta (Howell 1979; Lee 1979). Lee reports that a few Herero families began moving west in the 1920s. Because most land between the Delta and the Qangwa and Xai Xai valleys is virtually waterless, the expansion of Herero into this territory was sudden rather than gradual. Outside Ngamiland, there are large settlements of Herero at Rakops and Mahalapye and in the Ghanzi district.

Most of the Herero who survived the trek from South West Africa arrived in Bechuanaland empty handed. Not only did they leave behind their means of support, but most also lost the sacred pots, livestock, and fires of their ancestors. Those without cattle made a living by working as cattlehands for the few Herero who had livestock or by hiring themselves out to members of another tribe. Payment was typically in livestock, and by the 1920s they had accumulated enough cattle to become an independent ethnic group. Their economic success was accompanied by a resurgence of their ethnic identity. Many began rekindling the sacred fires of their ancestors and the national mark of lower tooth extraction came into use again.

While the Herero grew in economic prosperity, they did not increase in number. Accounts of Herero in South West Africa and Bechuanaland earlier in this century claimed that the Herero were a disappearing race, that they were 'committing tribal suicide' by limiting their fertility (Steenkamp 1944; Gibson 1959; Almagor 1982a). Our analyses of their fertility and mortality confirm Herero depopulation. The population of Herero appears to have been declining throughout most of the first half of this century (Chapter 10). Today, their demographic rates are similar to the rest of the people in Botswana.

History in Namibia

In Namibia and southern Angola there are peoples such as the Himba and Tjimba who share language, customs, and history with the Herero proper and Mbanderu in this study. In most historical accounts, the term *Tjimba* is applied to the hunter-gatherers and *Himba* to a separate group of pastoralists (van Warmelo 1962; Vedder 1966a; Vedder 1966b; Gibson 1952; Gibson 1977) living in the Kaokoveld. The Ovambo of northern Namibia and southern Angola have applied the term *Tjimba* to all branches of Herero, while the Herero proper and Mbanderu use *Tjimba* only to refer to their poor relatives in the Kaokoveld. Herero are also known as Damara in the literature and by many people in Southern Africa, although the term *Damara* is also applied to other groups in Namibia as well. There are also peoples such as the Vakwandu who speak Herero (Medeiros 1981) but who do not appear to be closely related to the other Herero speakers of Namibia and Botswana.

How the Herero came to occupy Namibia and how long they have been there are unknown, but they probably arrived in north-western Namibia during the sixteenth century and spread to central Namibia by the late eighteenth century. At the time of European contact in the nineteenth century, the Mbanderu, who are also known as eastern Herero, ranged roughly in the territory from Grootfontein to approximately 150 km south of Windhoek, extending east to what is now the Botswana border. The Herero proper occupied land west of this area. However, these boundaries shifted throughout the century in response to ongoing hostilities among the branches of Herero and between the Herero and neighbouring Nama, Ovambo, and Tswana peoples.

Most reconstructions of Herero origins are based on oral history. The reconstructions, however, are rarely in accord. Vedder (1966b) reconstructed the patrilineal genealogy of Chief Maharero back to the birth of Kengeza in 1530. Vedder's information suggests that Kengeza was a young man at the time of the migration to the Kaokoveld, placing the arrival of the Herero in Namibia at about 1550. In this monograph Vedder wrote that all Herero were originally called Mbanderu and that they came to the Kaokoveld through Tswana territory where they had been grazing their cattle. Hostilities broke out between some Mbanderu and Tswana, causing many Mbanderu to move west to the Kaokoveld. The group who left became the Herero proper while those who remained with the Tswana retained their identity as Mbanderu. Some of these Herero were unsuccessful at rearing cattle and turned to hunting and gathering. They became known as the Tjimba.

In an earlier publication, Vedder (1966a) speculated that Herero descended from the Hamite tribes of North Africa. He believed that philological evidence and references in Herero legends suggested that they had passed through the regions of the Central African lakes, from which they must have migrated west through southern Angola, turning south at the Atlantic Ocean, and crossing the Kunene River into the Kaokoveld. He also wrote that the name which the Herero call themselves, *Ovaherero*, means 'the people of yesterday'. He translated *Ovambanderu* as 'fighters of former times', and *Ovatjimba* is derived from 'Ondjimba', the Herero word for the African antbear. Vedder arrived at these definitions through linguistic and anecdotal inference. Unfortunately he made no attempt to reconcile the discrepancies between his two works.

In another account recorded from Mbanderu by Sundermeier (1986) it is written that the name *Ovambanderu* means 'people of the reeds', reflecting the nature of their original homeland. The Mbanderu said that they entered the Kaokoveld from the north, with the Kunene River always at their right-hand side. The Ovambo were the first to leave the place of the reeds and were later followed by the Herero proper and then the Mbanderu. While the Herero proper settled in the Kaokoveld, most of the Mbanderu moved further south and then dispersed in search of pasture. There are no suggested years for these migrations.

The arrival of Herero in central Namibia can be dated from the Sundermeier account. The Herero proper probably reached central Namibia around 1790 after the birth of Munjuku, who was the father of a prominent man named Kahimemua. Kahimemua is believed to have been born in the year *ojondjimanjakovindou*,[3] which was 1822 or 1823, so Munjuku was probably born around 1790. This date is supported by information

---

[3]Herero assigned names to each year, and the names have been aligned with years of the Gregorian calendar. The years of birth of most of the older people in our study were obtained this way. This system is described more fully in Chapter 2.

in Vedder (1966*b*), as 1790 is the year of birth reported for Tjamuaha, a contemporary of Munjuku. The arrival of Herero into central Namibia near the end of the eighteenth century is also supported by evidence in Vedder (1966*b*). He reports that Mutjise, who was the great grandfather of the great leader Maharero, left the Kaokoveld for the Okahandja area with a group of followers. Since Mutjise was born in 1730, and the movement appears to have occurred before his grandson Tjamuaha was a man, it is likely that the Herero proper moved into central Namibia late in the eighteenth century.

These accounts, though vague, suggest that branches of the Herero entered the Kaokoveld from either Botswana or Angola in about 1550 and occupied most of central Namibia by the nineteenth century. The most sensible explanation is that the Herero came from the Zambezi River area, entering Namibia from Angola in one or two migrations. That the first Herero migrants lived among the Tswana in north-western Botswana is unlikely, for Tswana did not occupy that territory until the nineteenth century (Tlou 1985). It is possible, however, that a group of Herero later migrated to Namibia through Botswana.

Bantu expansion into Southern Africa

The Khoisan, members of the language group that includes click sounds, are believed to have had exclusive occupation of Southern, central, and parts of eastern Africa until their territories were encroached upon by the expansion of Bantu and Cushitic peoples in East Africa about 3000 years ago (Ambrose 1982). It is believed that Khoisan have occupied Southern Africa for at least the last 24 000 years (Brooks 1989). It is generally accepted that Bantu began migrating east from West Africa, probably Cameroon (Greenberg 1963), at least 3000 years ago (Hall 1990) and possibly as long ago as 5000 years (Ehret 1982*a*). The routes of the migrations out of Cameroon and into central and Southern Africa are debated. Phillipson (1977) has argued that the Bantu moved both around and through the equatorial forest zone. One stream moved east and then south along the northern and western perimeters of the forest where they acquired Iron Age technology, cultivated grains and livestock. They converged with a western stream of Bantu that had moved through the forest to its south-western perimeter. Dispersal produced the south-western Bantu and, later, the south-eastern Bantu who brought Iron Age technology and food production to the Khoisan peoples already occupying the areas.

More recent archaeological and linguistic evidence indicates that food production in Southern Africa predates the arrival of Bantu (Deacon *et al.* 1978; Ehret 1982*b*; Hall 1990). Ehret also rejects the routes proposed by Phillipson, arguing that the linguistic evidence better supports a slow exodus of Bantu through the forests (Ehret 1982*b*) and that contact with the Iron Age and food producing people of the Central Sudan occurred from the forests.

Both scenarios place the spread of speakers of Herero-like languages (Western Highland group, south-western Bantu) from the south-western fringes of the forests into Angola and northern Namibia during the first millennium BC (Phillipson 1977; Ehret 1982*b*). Herero legends do not place their arrival there until more recently and suggest that they have been isolated for a long time, having only recently adopted pastoralism. The Herero words for cattle (*ozongombe*, sing. *ongombe*) appear to have Nilotic roots, suggesting that both the cattle and the cattle vocabulary were obtained from pastoralists of the middle Zambezi, who originally acquired their cattle from the north (Murdock 1959). Among the Bantu of south-eastern Africa, cattle vocabulary has been traced to Khoisan (Ehret 1967; Oliver and Fagan 1975; Ehret 1982*a*).

In sum, the historical, archaeological, and linguistic evidence to date suggests that the ancestors of Herero entered the savannah zone of south-western Africa from West Africa about 3000 years ago. Our historical information suggests that they did not enter northern Namibia until the sixteenth century, although other sources indicate that this occurred much earlier. Unlike other south-western Bantu tribes, Herero gave up horticulture altogether in favour of raising cattle (Murdock 1959). They must have arrived in Namibia as pastoralists only a few generations later. On their way to the Kaokoveld, the Herero may have herded cattle along the middle Zambezi, turning south between the Kunene and Okavango so that they would have entered the Kaokoveld with the Kunene at their 'right-hand side' as their own legends claim.

Biological approaches to history

Genetic markers are an independent source of information about Herero history, especially about their interactions with their neighbours. Marker studies indicate that the Herero have been isolated from their neighbours and that they have been a small population for a long time.

Heterozygosity

Harpending and Chasko (1976) studied heterozygosity at 17 loci in 15 Southern African populations and a pan-African sample. The original data were given in Nurse *et al.* (1978), Jenkins *et al.* (1978), and Jenkins (1972).

In a finite population, gene frequencies change through time because of genetic drift and gene flow. Genetic drift is sampling error from one generation to the next. The cumulative effect of drift is to reduce the diversity or heterozygosity of genes in the population. The smaller the group, the more rapid the loss of heterozygosity. Gene flow (mate exchange with other groups) restores heterozygosity. There are quite elaborate mathematical models of this process (Harpending and Ward 1982; Rogers and Harpending 1986) but they do not seem to provide much more insight into the meaning of real data than does the simple argument just given.

The 15 populations that Harpending and Chasko studied included five Bushman populations, one Damara[4] and two Khoi (Hottentot) groups, four Bantu-speaking peoples, and three South African and Namibian Coloured populations. They computed overall heterozygosity within each group, averaged over the 17 loci. These are listed in Table 1.1. There were highly significant differences among these groups.

Overall heterozygosity was lowest (0.259) in the most isolated Bushmen population in the sample, a group from a remote region on the border between Namibia and Botswana called /Du /Da. The five least heterozygous populations included three remote Bushmen groups, the Damara, and the Herero with heterozygosity of 0.281. There was a sensible progression from these apparently small or isolated groups to the Coloured population of Johannesburg with an average heterozygosity of 0.336. The other southern Bantu speakers in the sample, the Sotho and the Pedi, had average heterozygosities of 0.297–0.299.

The Herero, by this measure, were significantly either smaller or more isolated than other Bantu-speaking populations in the last several centuries. In this respect, they were similar to the other small isolated groups in northern Namibia and north-western Botswana today, like the Damara and the Bushmen. This is also their own view of their history. Herero origin myths that suggest descent from a few founders[5] and several centuries of autonomy in northern Namibia (Vedder 1966b) are supported by the genetic evidence.

Genetic distances

Genetic distance is a measure of dissimilarity between two sets of gene frequencies. Genetic distances among a set of populations determine a 'map' in the same sense that distances among cities on a road map determine the relative geometry of the cities. Of course a map of cities occupies two dimensions, but a map of genetic distances among n populations can occupy up to $n - 1$ dimensions. A standard data reduction technique, principal components analysis, can produce a two-dimensional representation of the $n - 1$ dimensions to make it more comprehensible.

Harpending and Jenkins (1973) used principal components to compute

---

[4]The term *Damara* in this section refers to a people also known in Namibia as 'Black Bushmen'. They are dark-skinned people who lived by hunting and gathering in northern Namibia and speak a Khoisan language.

[5]The Herero say that they descended from six original mothers, after whom their matrilineages are named. The Herero lineage system is discussed in the last section of this chapter.

Table 1.1. Heterozygosity at 17 loci in a sample of African populations. The Bushmen populations are all speakers of the !Kung or northern Bush language except the Naron, who speak central Bush. 'Africans' is a pseudopopulation, a collection of marker frequencies from Cavalli-Sforza and Bodmer (1971) from various groups in Africa

Population	Heterozygosity	Standard Error
/Du /Da Bushmen, Botswana	0.259	0.007
Naron Bushmen, Ghanzi, Botswana	0.263	0.008
Damara, northern Namibia	0.264	0.008
Xai Xai Bushmen, Botswana	0.274	0.006
Herero Bantu, Botswana	0.281	0.009
Dobe Bushmen, Botswana	0.286	0.003
Sesfontein Khoi, Namibia	0.288	0.009
Kau Kau Bushmen, Botswana	0.288	0.005
Sotho (Group A) Bantu, South Africa	0.297	0.008
Pedi Bantu, South Africa	0.297	0.005
Kuboes Coloured, Namibia	0.299	0.005
Africans, pan-Africa	0.299	0.005
Sotho (Group B) Bantu, South Africa	0.299	0.007
Keetmanshoop Khoi, Namibia	0.308	0.005
Sesfontein Coloured, South Africa	0.336	0.007
Johannesburg Coloured, South Africa	0.336	0.006

such a genetic distance map of 18 populations from Southern Africa. The two-dimensional representation accounted for 58 per cent of the dispersion of the 18 points. This means that the two-dimensional map is a very good portrayal of the complicated 17-dimensional swarm.

All the Bushmen populations were clustered together, meaning that they were very similar to each other. Another clear cluster was formed by the Bantu populations along with the Damara, the Khoi, and the Coloured groups from Sesfontein in Namibia. A third loose cluster was composed of Khoi and Coloured groups from South Africa and southern Namibia. Adding a third dimension to the map, again using principal components analysis, led to a picture that accounted for 70 per cent of the actual dispersion. The third dimension showed that the Khoi, Coloured, and Damara populations of Sesfontein were quite distinct from the Bantu-speaking groups, though there was some similarity in the two-dimensional representation.

The Herero in this study were the least like the Khoi of all the Bantu groups. The genetic data suggested no substantial gene exchange with any of their Khoisan-speaking neighbours (either Bushmen, Khoi, or Damara) in the northern Kalahari. Their closest Bantu-speaking relatives were

Bantu from Mozambique, on the other side of the continent, and the Swazi from South Africa. There were no other south-western Bantu in the study. A later similar study (Nurse *et al.* 1985) based on a larger set of markers found the same patterns. This latter study included the Ovambo and other Bantu-speaking groups from northern Namibia. As expected, the Herero were genetically similar to these neighbours, with whom they also share linguistic and cultural traits.

Mitochondrial typing

Vigilant *et al.* (1991), report DNA sequences of two hypervariable segments of the control region of mitochondria from 189 people, including 121 native Africans.

Most people in the sample had a mitochondrial DNA sequence that was not shared with anyone else in the sample: there were 135 distinct types in the sample of 189 people. The sample of 189 people included 27 Herero, and of these 27 Herero, 19 possessed an identical mitochondrial type! This implies that the Herero have an unusually low level of mitochondrial diversity, although the mitochondria in the other 8 Herero in the sample were quite different from the common one. This reduced diversity is probably the signature of a severe bottleneck within the last few millennia.

Fig. 1.4 shows these patterns in the mitochondria of more recent, larger samples of !Kung and Herero. These are distributions of the number of differences (i) out of approximately 700 sites between all possible pairs of mitochondria. The solid lines are theoretical curves derived in Rogers and Harpending (1992). Most pairs of Herero mitochondria are identical ($i=0$) or else differ at only a few sites, while the distribution of differences between !Kung mitochondria has a wave-like form with a peak at 10–11 differences. Rogers and Harpending show that the Herero pattern reflects a population bottleneck within the last several hundred years. The wave in the !Kung mitochondrial difference distribution appears in other human populations. It is the signature of an ancient population expansion, about 50 000–100 000 years ago. Rogers and Harpending use the position of this wave peak to date the origins of anatomically modern humans.

The mitochondrial sequences show that the several tens of thousands of Herero in Namibia and Botswana today are derived from a very few mothers in the recent past, in agreement with their own view of the origins of their matrilineages. Their origin is so recent that it is impossible to date it with real confidence using current population genetic methods but it is certainly within the last millennium.

Summary of marker studies

Linguistic data indicate that south-western Bantu languages became established earlier than the languages spoken by south-eastern Bantu (Phillipson

Herero

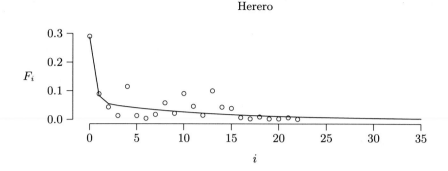

!Kung

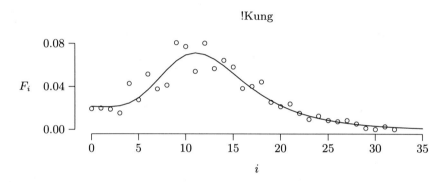

Fig. 1.4. Mitochondrial difference distributions of Herero and !Kung. The distributions show the number of differences between all possible pairs of mitochondria. The Herero pattern shows that the population underwent a recent bottleneck, while the !Kung distribution shows the wave that is the signature of the ancient population expansion of anatomically modern humans. These figures were calculated from unpublished data of Himla Soodyall, Trefor Jenkins, Linda Vigilant, Margaret Gregowicz, and Stephen Sherry. The model was fit and the figure provided by Alan Rogers.

1977). In addition, the similarities among the south-eastern Bantu languages indicate that the spread into south-eastern Africa was rapid. The genetic data support these interpretations, but other interpretations are possible. The south-eastern Bantu populations show a much higher level of heterozygosity and smaller genetic distances among themselves than the south-western Bantu, indicating that they share a more recent common ancestor than the group of south-western Bantu. However, heterozygosity becomes lower and genetic distance becomes larger more quickly in small populations, and we believe the effect of small population sizes may be an important factor.

Infertility and population history

Nurse *et al.* (1985, p. 149) remark, 'It is not easy to understand why, if there were population pressures in central Angola at the beginning of the present era, it should not have been until fifteen hundred years later that the Iron Age came to Namibia'. What, they are asking, accounts for the low density and fragmented ethnicity of Bantu-speaking people of this western part of Southern Africa. We suggest that pathological sterility may be the missing part of this puzzle, that the Herero and others have been in the region a long time and that they have either been declining or hovering around stationarity for centuries while the Bantu expansion in the east was not affected. Today, the African infertility belt starts in the south-west with the Herero and probably the !Kung and extends north-eastward to the Sudan. It is not reported in the south-east where the great expansions, wars, and upheavals of the eighteenth and nineteenth centuries occurred.

The issue of historically low Herero fertility and the 'African infertility belt' is dealt with explicitly in more detail throughout this book, but especially in Chapters 5 and 6. Our data extending back to the latter decades of the nineteenth century indicate that Herero have experienced pathologically low fertility (probably caused by sexually-transmitted diseases) since before the turn of the century. The older Herero women we interviewed averaged less than four births each, and our indirect estimates of the fertility of women living a generation earlier indicate that they also had few births. A number of scholars have argued that African sub-fertility must be recent because depopulation would have resulted otherwise. How far back pathological sub-fertility has persisted in Africa we cannot say, but, given that the genetic data suggest a period of long isolation, a long history is possible. If the Bantu in this region have suffered from sub-fertility since their arrival there, the proposed routes of the Bantu migrations must take this into account. How, for example, did south-western Bantu peoples come into contact with diseases that the south-eastern peoples either avoided or mitigated? The diseases probably entered sub-Saharan Africa from the north, where they have been known since at least Biblical times (see Chapter 6).

One possibility described by Ehret (1982*a*) is that the southern equatorial savannah was occupied by Khoisan-speaking pastoralists when the Bantu arrived. A major weakness in this scenario, however, is that the south-western Bantu, including the Herero, have essentially no Khoisan ancestry, as expected from incidental contact between peoples living in the same region. In contrast, south-eastern Bantu speakers have from 15 to 60 per cent Khoisan ancestry.

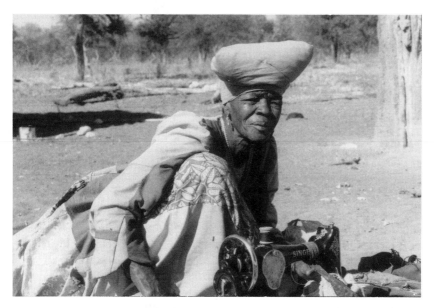

Fig. 1.5. Herero woman sewing distinctive Victorian dress. Cloth for the dresses are purchased in local shops.

Life in Botswana

Way of life

The Herero are self-consciously ethnic, and there is today almost no marriage with members of other groups. Adult women wear distinctive Victorian dresses (see Fig. 1.5) that stand out so that they are prominent and visible in much the same way that Amish or Mennonites are visible in rural areas of the north-eastern United States or that Orthodox Jews are visible in New York City.

For two or three decades following the war, however, Herero ethnicity seemed forgotten. Many worked for the Tawana (northern Tswana), and others were converted to Christianity. In the 1920s, when Herero had acquired enough cattle to leave Tawana employment and live off their own herds, there was a resurgence of their own traditions. Circumcision and tooth extraction came into practice again, and the missionaries lost their converts as Herero began rekindling the sacred fires of their ancestors. Today, they are considered wealthy cattle herders and staunch traditionalists by other ethnic groups in Botswana.

Although more than 35 years have passed, Gibson's 1953 work among Herero in Botswana still accurately depicts the way of life of most of them today (see Gibson 1956, 1959). A more recent account of the Herero proper can also be found in the monograph by Vivelo (1977). The best English summary of Herero life before the Herero–German War is in Vedder (1966a). An excellent summary of Vedder's account and most of the early German sources is in Gibson (1952). We recommend consulting these sources for more detailed ethnographic descriptions of Herero, while Vedder (1966b), Gibson (1962), Almagor (1980; 1982b; 1982a), Poewe (1985), and Alnaes (1989) may be useful for dealing with more specific topics. A history of the Mbanderu tribe in their own words is in Sundermeier (1986).

The theme of loss of traditional ways is prominent in the older literature about the Herero, and it is prominent in conversations with older people. On the other hand the customs that we observed were much the same as those described in the nineteenth century. Old people complain that the holy fires are not kept, but there are holy fires everywhere. The most emphatic and articulate statement of distress about the loss of Herero customs that we heard concerned milking into a metal container rather than a wooden bowl. The target of this complaint, however, was a neighbour of our informant, who was one of the wealthier women in the area, and the context of the conversation was not, it seemed, abstract evaluation of the tribal way of life.

Subsistence

Like the Namibian homeland, the northern Kalahari is a harsh environment. Descriptions of other populations living there suggest that it offers barely enough to eke out a living. The !Kung, for example, have lived marginally in this environment as hunter-gatherers (Chapter 9). The Herero appear to have fared much better economically, specializing in goat and cattle husbandry, in competition with the Tswana, most of whom practice mixed (livestock and crop) farming, and with other agricultural and riverine groups such as the Kgalagadi, Yei, and Mbukushu. In Botswana, the richest are those who own the most cattle (Litschauer and Kelly 1981), and nearly all Herero either have a few cattle of their own or can depend on kinsmen in times of need.

Although we do not have good estimates of the number of cattle that the average Herero owns, per capita livestock ownership is higher in Ngamiland than in most other parts of the country (Litschauer and Kelly 1981). Overall per capita income is higher in Botswana than in most other sub-Saharan African nations (Lesetedi et al. 1989). Much of the current wealth in cattle may be due to favourable terms of trade with the European Economic Community (Peters 1986), but the Herero are clearly successful at their subsistence strategy and have been for years. Moreover, livestock has been a major export of Botswana for several decades (May and McLellan 1971; Mitchell 1982; Peters 1986).

In 1980 the Ngamiland district of Botswana contained 354 000 head

Table 1.2. Cattle counts in the Dobe region veterinary department crushes, 1982 to 1988

Date	Xai Xai	Xubi	Magopa	Baate	Qangwa	Xgoshe	Total
4/82	589	638	1481	440	1714	1648	6510
8/82	718	569	1514	607	1172	1395	5975
4/83	720	670	1505	524	1488	1028	5935
8/83	707	645	1103	925	942	844	5166
4/84	878	717	1532	682	1021	698	5528
8/84	1011	730	1274	386	954	909	5264
4/85	1011	1272	1493	493	973	1043	6285
8/85	1137	678	1364	477	825	1051	5532
4/86	796	661	1735	549	948	972	5661
4/87	864	671	1850	553	1338	1211	6487
8/87	977	641	1467	429	1227	1005	5746
4/88	694	540	1925	453	1223	744	5579

of cattle according to the 1980 *Agricultural survey* (Litschauer and Kelly 1981) carried out by the Ministry of Agriculture. The 1981 census (Central Statistics Office 1981) enumerated 68 000 people in Ngamiland so there were slightly more than five head of cattle per person in this district. Much of this herd is owned by Herero, who constitute perhaps 10 per cent of the population of Ngamiland. Since ethnic affiliation is not recorded by government agencies in Botswana, there are no data available about Herero stock ownership *per se* in official statistics. However, we can estimate per capita ownership for the Qangwa–Xai Xai region of western Ngamiland and compare this with information published by other authors who have tallied population and cattle counts for Herero areas.

The Qangwa and Xai Xai valleys are a region well known to anthropologists as the 'Dobe area' in studies of !Kung Bushmen carried out by the Harvard Kalahari Project (Lee and DeVore 1976). Surrounded by waterless uninhabited desert, these valleys together are a defined closed area where we have complete enumeration of Herero speakers as well as data from 1968 given in Lee (1979).

We counted 387 Herero in this area in 1987, a number that should not be taken too literally given the high mobility of individuals. Lee reported that there were 350 'Blacks' in this region in 1968: perhaps 50 of these were members of other Bantu-speaking groups such as the Tawana and the Yei. Lee also reported that there were 4500 head of cattle here, almost all of them owned by Herero and other Bantu-speakers. There were thus 13 cattle per person in 1968, if only a few these cattle were owned by any of the 400 or so !Kung who also lived there.

Table 1.2 shows unpublished counts of cattle recorded by the Botswana veterinary department during twice yearly vaccination campaigns in 1982 through 1988. Each veterinary cattle crush serves many homesteads in the area. The crushes for which data are given in the table serve established Herero, Tswana, and Yei communities—crushes that serve new boreholes on the periphery of the region are not included since these are owned by absentee Tswana, not by local Herero.

The number of cattle in the region, shown as the total in the last column, is about 6000 head with considerable variation from year to year. This variation reflects movement of cattle in and out of the area, the offtake of cattle to market that occurs in the winter before the August round of vaccination, and occasionally missing herds that have wandered away and were taken to different crushes.

Some of these cattle belong to members of other ethnic groups, and we can guess that they are the property of 450 people, the 387 Herero that we counted in the region and 63 members of other tribes, to estimate that there are 6000/450 or 13.3 head of cattle per person. This is two and a half times the per capita cattle density of Ngamiland as a whole, and it is very close to the figure of 13 head per person reported by Lee.

Gibson (1962) presents data on stock in the Sehitwa area (by Lake Ngami) in 1952. There were 28 605 head of cattle and an estimated 5000 people in the area, of whom 1000–1500 were probably Herero. The other people in the area invest more in gardens and goats and less in cattle than do the Herero. If there were 1000 Herero in the Sehitwa region in 1952, and if half the cattle belonged to Herero, then there were 14 head of cattle per Herero, which is consistent with our estimates from the Dobe region.

Wagner (1957) describes Herero economics in the Otjimbingue Reserve in South West Africa. The 544 Herero on the reserve owned 3100 head of cattle. This *per capita* cattle density of 5.7 is less than half that of Herero in Ngamiland, but the situation at Otjimbingue may have been transient. There was a severe drought in 1946, after which the total number of head was 1644. This includes cattle owned by members of other groups as well as by Herero. By 1951 there were 4268 cattle on the reserve, and even this number may have been below the long term equilibrium cattle population of the reserve.

In 1972, cattle holdings among Herero speakers of the north-western Kaokoveld was estimated at 12 per capita (Malan 1974). This is the same herd density per capita that we observed in Ngamiland.

Besides cattle, Herero also depend on goats, which are more drought resistant than cattle, sheep, and other livestock for subsistence. Many also own chickens, donkeys, horses, dogs, and cats. The Herero's preferred food is sour milk, but they also purchase large quantities of food from stores. Heavily sugared tea with milk and corn meal and samp, which were frequently made into porridges and flavoured with sour milk and meat when they were available, were staples. Excepting important occasions, cattle were rarely slaughtered by their owners to be eaten. In the bush, however, it was not infrequent that a cow would be wounded by a predator or fall in a well and be available for consumption. Some larger villages had 'meat trees', from which partially butchered carcasses of cattle or goats were hung and sold by the chunk.

Herero also collect a few bush foods, especially during drought years. Most families plant crops such as maize, sorghum, melons, and sugar cane, but these often fail and are probably not an important source of subsistence for most Herero. In 1988, we noticed that most gardens in the Magopa region produced poor yields, while to the north at Nxau Nxau some gardens were quite successful. Many gardens, including those that failed, were quite large, probably encompassing several tens of thousand square feet as shown in Fig. 1.6(a). A substantial amount of work is required to establish these gardens, as the fields had to be cleared and enclosed with thorn brush fences to keep out cattle and goats. Typically, the large gardens were cleared and fenced by several members of a homestead, each having his own area within the field to plant. Many gardens were simply small enclosures behind huts in the homestead, but some of them, such as the one in Fig. 1.6(b), were quite productive.

Herero obtain most of their cash through sale of cattle to the Botswana Meat Commission. A few, particularly men, are engaged in wage employment in the larger towns of Botswana and in Namibia, but it is unlikely that these wage earners provide an important economic base for the Herero living at the remote villages and cattleposts in this study; few Herero were reported by relatives to be away working, although many Herero had at some point in their life been employed. Although they are in many respects self-sufficient, most Herero need cash to purchase clothing and household and farm goods.

The homestead

Herero live in extended family homesteads called *ozonganda* (sing. *onganda*). An *onganda* is ideally a patrilineal unit composed of one or more huts along with goat and cattle kraals. The *onganda* is headed by a senior male and includes his wife or wives, his sons and their wives and children, and his unmarried daughters and their children. Other relatives such as brothers but especially unmarried sisters and their children may also live in the *onganda*. The head of an *onganda* is responsible for its members, who are expected to consult him before acting on important matters. If the patrilineage possesses the holy fire of their *oruzo*, then the head of the *onganda* has official duties resembling those of a priest.

Although the *ozonganda* are theoretically patrilineal units, in practice

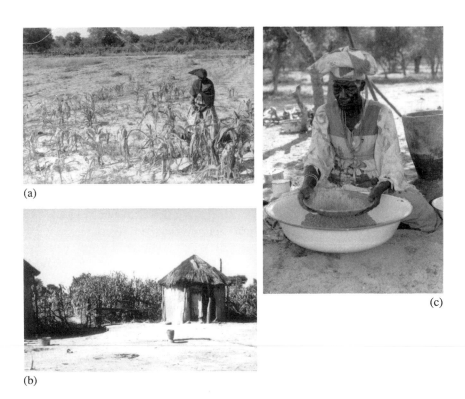

(a)

(b)

(c)

Fig. 1.6. Herero fields and gardens. (a) Large fields in the Magopa region showed poor yields in 1987–8. (b) Small garden enclosures behind huts, such as this one in Sehitwa, were sometimes quite productive. The hut is on the verge of collapse due to heavy rain in 1988–9. (c) This Herero woman is sorting produce from her garden.

they are often matrilineal for several reasons. Women leave their natal *onganda* at marriage, but the frequency of divorce, Herero and spousal death prompts many women to return to their matrilineal kinsmen. In old age, when the homesteads become dominated by the offspring of brothers, women will return to the homestead of their sons. Thus, a typical homestead we observed was centred on the senior male, his mother, his brothers, and his sisters and their children. The sons of a polygynous senior male frequently fissioned into separate *ozonganda* following the death of their father. The descendants of each mother formed the cores of the new *ozonganda*. This was also described by Gibson (1956).

The huts of the *onganda* are usually round mud dwellings measuring no more than 10 feet in diameter and roofed with grass. The preferred mortar is composed of dung from cattle and earth from termite hills. The wall structure is formed of poles set upright in a circle. These are filled from the inside and out with mud plaster. Many prefer to build square houses and top them with aluminum siding, and a few have built huts from concrete bricks purchased at a quarry. The doorway is usually purchased from a shop. Many also buy beds and other furniture for them. Huts are built by women over the course of three or four months, but men may assist from time to time by gathering some building materials or by sawing poles. Properly maintained, these huts may last for several decades. Several Herero huts in various stages of construction are shown in Fig. 1.7.

The average number of huts in 29 Herero homesteads we surveyed around Lake Ngami was 3.6 with a standard deviation (SD) of 2.5 huts, the largest homestead having 12 huts.[6] The huts are small, averaging 10.5 m^2 in area (SD=3.8, $n = 38$). Our census of the huts belonging to 39 women (most men sleep in the huts of their wives or mothers) we interviewed near the end of the rainy season in 1989 shows that 2.5 people occupy the average Herero hut (SD=2.7). Our estimate is lower than the estimate reported in the 1981 Botswana census (Central Statistics Office 1987), which counted dwelling or household units for the denominator rather than number of huts. If we count multiple huts owned by women as a single dwelling unit, we estimate that there are 4.3 persons per Herero dwelling unit.

Most activity takes place in the *onganda* yard so that huts are mainly used for sleeping and storage of belongings. Most Herero cook over open fires using wood collected by women. In the larger villages, water for domestic consumption can be obtained from government boreholes, but in most areas of this study it is collected from hand-dug wells or from pools of water left from the rain. Women transport water by the bucketful on their heads. Larger quantities of water may be loaded in small plastic drums onto the backs of donkeys, while large steel drums full of water are rolled by hand or towed by livestock back to the homestead. Women perform all domestic duties such as cooking, milking, fetching water, washing clothes, caring for children, and collecting firewood while men are responsible for tending livestock. When they are not at school, girls may help with domestic tasks while boys may help look after livestock. Both cattle and goats are milked. The milk of cows may be drunk fresh, but it is usually manufactured into sour milk in calabashes, and the fat is used to make butter (see Fig. 1.8).

Apart from milking, most of the labour involved in livestock management is restricted to providing water for the animals during the dry season. Compared to other African pastoral groups, such as the Turkana (Gulliver 1955), cattle are not closely watched and herding is not a central activity of boys. Vivelo (1977) described Herero cattle management as *laissez-faire*.

---

[6]We defined a hut as any building with a roof that was not abandoned.

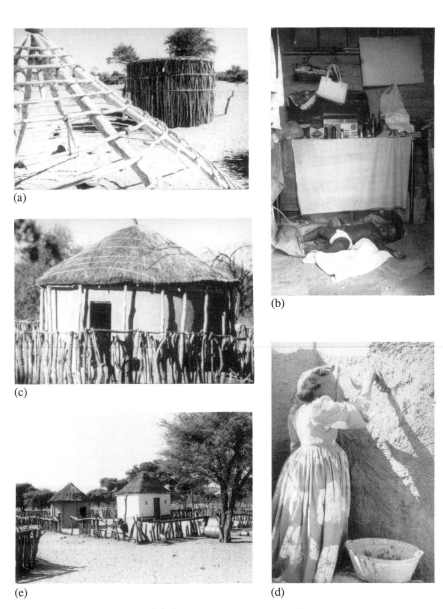

Fig. 1.7. Herero huts. (a) A partially constructed hut. The roof frame is in the foreground. (b) Inside a brick hut. Huts built with modern and traditional materials are both well furnished. (c) A classic round hut. (d) A Herero woman plastering her hut with a mud–cow dung mixture. (e) A traditional and a fancy square hut. The fence around the two huts encloses a 'female household' within the homestead, as the huts are owned by a single woman.

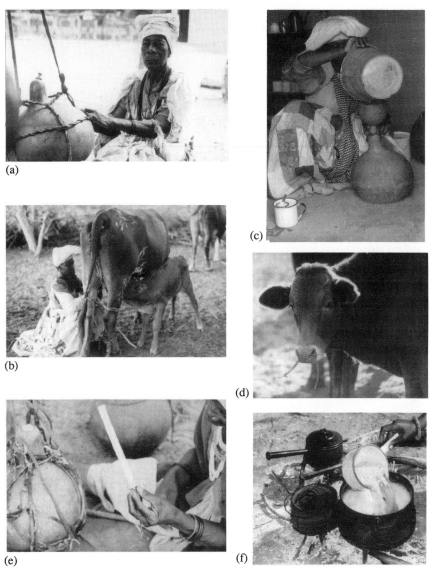

Fig. 1.8. Milking and preparation of dairy products. (a) Herero woman shaking calabash to make skim milk. (b) Calf competing for its mother's milk. The calf is allowed to suckle while its mother is milked. The cow's legs are tied to to prevent it from running away and kicking during milking. (c) Woman pouring fresh milk into calabash. (d) Calf with weaning twigs in nostrils. Herero also place aluminum cans on the ends of calves' noses when they 'refuse to be weaned'. (e) The clumping of fat on the calabash plug indicates when the milk is ready. (f) Preparation of Herero fat (*omaze*). Butter from milk is cooked until it changes to *omaze*, which Herero say can still be eaten years later.

Although calves are corralled, the remainder of the herd is free to wander and graze during the night. Cows with calves turn up in the morning to feed their young during which time they are also milked by women. Some Herero keep the mothers of their calves in a separate corral during the night and move them into the calves' corral when it is time for milking. Calves are allowed to suckle on one teat while milk from the other is squeezed into a pail. During the day, Herero males ride on donkey or horseback to check on their herds but do not spend the day watching over them. Livestock are lost to predators such as lions, hyenas, and, occasionally, Cape dogs. Some also die from eating the toxic weed *otjikuriama* (*Dychopetalum cymosum*).

Apparently cattle theft is not a major problem. The beasts belonging to an *onganda* are branded alike while individuals earmark them to identify personal ownership. Herding is more important during the rainy season than during the dry season. Abundant grass and water pans allow the herd to disperse so that cattle are more likely to be lost. Herds are moved when the pans dry up or when the grass has been eaten away. After the pans disappear, cattle collect around man-made wells where they are fed water by the bucketful as shown in Fig. 1.9. The end of the dry season coincides with the hottest part of the year, and men may spend several hours a day in the hot sun lifting water for their livestock. A few Herero homesteads around Sehitwa had diesel generated pumps, but most Herero are reluctant to invest in these (Almagor 1982*b*).

We do not understand completely the division of labour in Herero homesteads. Part of the problem is that anthropologists are accustomed to examining economic productivity at the household level. Defining what makes up a Herero household is complex. There seem to be two independent spheres of household management. On one level there is livestock management at the *onganda* level known as the 'farming household' (Peters 1986). This is the domain of men. When and if a woman marries she may initially bring only a few of her cattle to her new homestead. If the marriage endures, over time more of her cattle will be brought from the herd of her father or brothers to the herd of her husband's homestead. This means that a man may be simultaneously managing not only his own cattle, but the cattle of his wives, his sisters, his mother and their children as well as other dependents.

Household management also takes place on a smaller level, which is also the level of consumption. Within the homestead are individual domestic units managed by women. Women own separate huts or clusters of huts within the *onganda*, and their is little overlap in responsibilities. Co-wives prepare separate pots of food and feed and clothe their children separately. Both men and women own livestock, and cash from their sale and their produce (such as milk) is controlled by the owner. Men may divert their resources to their wives, to other kinsmen, and to girlfriends. Within a

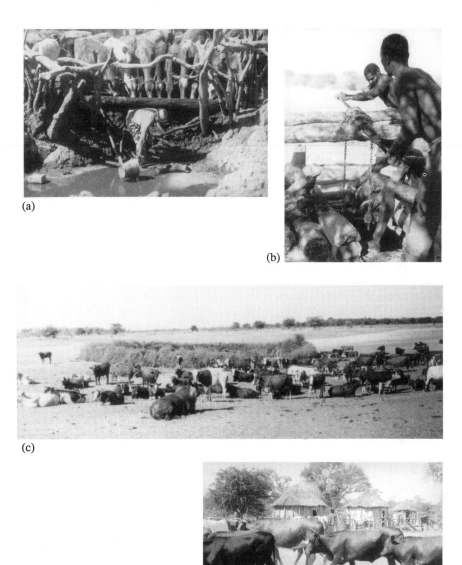

Fig. 1.9. Watering and tending cattle. (a) Old man lifting water for cattle from shallow well. (b) Two or three men are required to lift water from crank wells. (c) Cattle and other livestock wait at the well to be watered. The well is enclosed within a brush fence. (d) Cattle wander untended from the corral to the well.

homestead there may be economic heterogeneity. People may belong to more than one homestead and move among them freely. Yet, an individual's wealth depends on successful management of the herd. Because each sex may have competing goals, it is difficult to discuss what a household is at either level.

We also do not have a clear understanding of the biological importance of sexual division of labour nor even of marriage (see Chapter 7). Our impression is that women work more hours than men but expend less energy. A glance at a homestead reveals clusters of sessile women who appear to be doing little or nothing. Milking in the morning and evening requires roughly half an hour a day. Younger women may be engaged in hut construction but the other tasks of women such as cooking and child-care may involve only directing the activities of older children. Other female tasks such as fetching water and firewood, washing clothes, and processing food consume substantial time and energy.

The work of men, however, seems more strenuous and risky. In the wet season cattle are dispersed widely over the landscape and are tended, moved, and monitored by men. In the dry season and during drought years, as the wells dry up, watering cattle requires long hours in the full sun lifting water to fill the troughs. Several men that we knew were killed by lions while protecting the herds (see Fig. 1.10), and there are other perils like falling in wells.

Double descent and lineage

Paternal descent

Herero trace descent bilaterally, that is, through their mothers and their fathers. Through his father, every Herero acquires his (or her) *oruzo* (pl. *otuzo*). If a child's mother is unmarried and the child's father does not claim him, the child takes the *oruzo* of his mother's father. A woman adopts the *oruzo* of her husband at marriage. A man may claim the children he has with an unmarried girlfriend through payment of cattle to the family of the girlfriend. The transfer of cattle gives the father legal paternal rights in his children, though the children's status may be junior to that of the father's marital children. These 'purchased' children adopt their father's *oruzo* once they have been claimed.

The *otuzo* have been called patriclans, but they appear to be religious rather than social groups. They prescribe customs such as what foods individuals may not eat and what colour cattle they should keep. They are patrilineal because membership in them is primarily based on paternal descent and because the livestock and paraphernalia of an *oruzo* are inherited patrilineally. Associated with each of them are special herds of cattle and vessels such as wooden milking pails to be used for cows of a

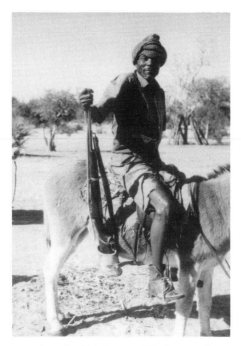

Fig. 1.10. Man preparing for lion hunt. We knew of several men who were killed or wounded by lions in the course of a hunt.

particular lineage (see Fig. 1.11). Each *oruzo* also has a holy fire, which is the centre of most religious activities. The holy fire (Fig. 1.11 is owned by the head of the patriclan and maintained by his senior wife. Before the Herero–German War, the *otuzo* were widely practiced and respected but have since fallen into disuse, at least in Botswana. Although there are holy fires everywhere, many Herero did not know their *otuzo*, and those who did frequently disregarded them without fear. In contrast, Vedder (1966a) wrote that Herero, when offered meat, would inquire carefully about the appearance of the beast before eating it.

In our interviews we asked people to provide the names of the *otuzo* of themselves and their family members. A list of 22 *otuzo* we heard about is given in Table 1.3. Our list may be compared to the list found in Gibson (1952), which was based on a summary of secondary sources, and to the discussion in Gibson (1956). Although some *otuzo* are unique to only the Mbanderu or Herero proper, our list is compiled from *otuzo* named by members of both tribes. Our impression is that many names for *otuzo* we heard about were actually different names for the same set of customs. For example, most people named their *otuzo* by referring to their prescriptions.

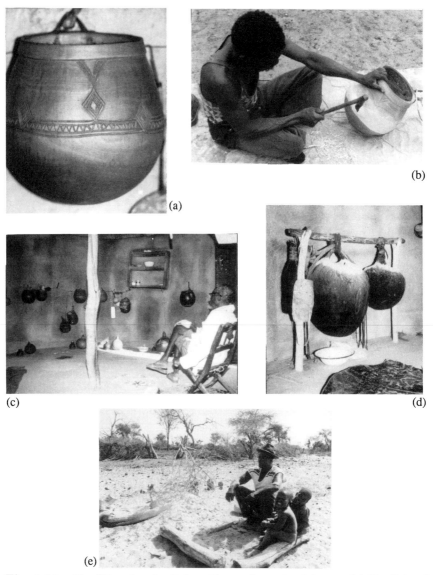

Fig. 1.11. Traditional and religious Herero homestead items. (a) Traditional wooden milking pail. (b) Man carving wooden pail. (c) Old man sitting in the great house with his ancestral vessels. Many of these vessels were brought from Namibia during the Herero–German War. (d) Skins for storing Herero fat (see Fig. 1.8) inside the great house. (e) Herero man with his two male heirs by his holy fire. The holy fire is the upside down brush. The cattle corral is in the background.

Table 1.3. List of Herero and Mbanderu *otuzo*

Omuko, Etumbo	Omuhinaruzo	Otjihaviria, Ombuindja
Okanene	Esembi, Onganjimi	Onguakavero
Omakoti	Ohorongo	Otjiporo
Ohambandarua	Ombongoro	Otjitjindua
Okoto	Onguatjia	Ongueuva
Onguendjandje	Otjirungu	Ondjiva
Ondanga	Otjiseu	Onguangoro
Onguatjindua		

Since an *oruzo* can have more than one prescription, it may be referred to in more than one way. Despite our efforts we were unable to clarify all of the discrepancies. However, we were able to conclude with a fair amount of confidence that a number or terms refer to the same *oruzo*; these equivalences are indicated in our list. Since a Herero adopts both his or her surname and *oruzo* from his or her social father, all who descended from the same paternal line should have the same *oruzo*. By cross-checking surnames with *otuzo*, we were able to determine, for example, that *omuko* and *etumbo* actually refer to the same customs. Several Herero confirmed this conclusion. Several also told us that *omuhinaruzo* (of the Marenga clan, which means literally, 'a person without an *oruzo*') is the same as the *ongueuva oruzo* of the Murangi clan. However, this claim was vehemently denied by others. One of our informants told us that *otjihaviria* is the Mbanderu term and *onguatjia* is the Herero proper term for identical sets of customs, but we were unable to find enough Herero proper and Mbanderu belonging to either *oruzo* to verify this.

While we attempt no analysis of the patrilineal groups, the *otuzo* are of interest because they identify paternal descent groups. The correspondence between patrilineage and biology is not perfect, however, since a child born out of wedlock adopts the patrilineage of his or her mother's father. Further error is introduced by weak paternity confidence.

The lack of strong patrilineal practices among Herero may reflect the loss of many sacred ancestral cattle and sacred vessels and neglect of the holy fires during the flight from the Germans. Even so, the *otuzo* have not been abandoned altogether. Many Herero would defer to their *otuzo* when asked for reasons for their peculiar behaviour. Other customs have also persisted, for example, circumcision of males and tooth extraction of two of the lower incisors among adolescents.

Many Herero have chosen to combine Herero customs with Christianity. One of the most traditional Mbanderu we knew conducted Sunday worship services from the Bible. He was in Israel during the Second World War and believes that the candles that he observed in cathedrals in southern Europe correspond to the holy fires of the Herero. Many Herero have learned to read from a Herero translation of the Bible distributed by the Lutheran Church.

Maternal descent

Every Herero is born into the *eanda* (pl. *omaanda*) of his or her mother, which is retained throughout life, regardless of marriage or paternity claims. According to legend, all Herero descended from the daughters of one mother; the descendants of each of these daughters form the lineages of each *eanda*, which takes its name from the founding daughter. Within each house there are subdivisions (see Gibson 1952), but not all Herero were familiar with these, although every Herero knows his or her *eanda*. In our field-work, an individual identified him or herself as either *omukueuva, omukuenambura, omukuendata, omukuatjivi, omukuatjiti, omukuaoti, omukuendjandje* or *omukuahera*.

In earlier sources (see Gibson 1952), *omukuahere* was interpreted to be a subhouse of *omukuendjandje*, and *omukuatjiti* was a subhouse of *omukuaoti* such that there were only six rather than eight *omaanda*. Several Herero we met, however, objected to this interpretation, saying that they are all daughters of the same mother and constitute separate *eanda*. Whatever their origin, there are clearly eight major *omaanda* today. An *eanda* does not appear to be associated with any special obligations or customs, such as food taboos or special observations of ancestors. But because every Herero knows his *eanda*, the *omaanda* are clearly very important.

In casual conversations one of the first pieces of information new acquaintances exchanged was their *omaanda*. Members of the same *eanda* consider each other kin, and may call each other brother or sister, regardless of tribal affinities. In the past, the *omaanda* were associated with herds of cattle distinct from the cattle of the *otuzo*. These cattle were passed to subsequent lines through matrilineal descent. In Botswana, however, inheritance of wealth is legally patrilineal such that the structure of Herero social organization may have been seriously disrupted, or at least many Herero men claim this is so.

Marriage and kinship

The preferred marriage of a Herero man is a cross-cousin of his father's *eanda*, especially his father's sister's daughter. Herero told us that marriage is exogamous with respect to *omaanda* but that marriage between members of the same *oruzo* is not prohibited.[7] In practice exogamy is not strictly followed. Marriages between members of the same *eanda* occurred in 12

---

[7]But see Schapera (1945), who reports that marriage should be exogamous in both lineages.

per cent (90/743) of the marriages we recorded. Schapera (1945) also found that 17 per cent of the marriages he recorded were between members of the same *eanda*. If we take into account the numbers of Herero belonging to various *omaanda* in these marriages, the frequency of endogamy would be about 20 per cent if spouses of each *eanda* were chosen at random. While the Herero are not strictly exogamous, they appear to make some effort to avoid intermarrying.

We also found that about 55 per cent (165/301) of the men for whom we had all the needed data married women of their fathers' *omaanda*, again suggesting that matrilineage is an important factor in marriage arrangements. One function of these marriage rules may be to ensure that a man's grandchildren will inherit his cattle, albeit through the progeny of his daughters. Informal inquiry about current inheritance practices suggests that the rules are not as simple as have been described. For example, informants agree that children of unmarried women inherit nothing from the biological father, even if the father has purchased rights in the child. Yet at the distribution of cattle following the death of young man we knew, the (paternal) relatives responsible for the disposition of the herd allocated animals to relatives of all degree, including an unacknowledged daughter by a !Kung mother.

We made a few attempts to account for the ownership of cattle belonging to individuals and learned that many had already been given away, although these individuals still have control over the beasts. Several informants told us that the reason old women have more cattle than old men is that, during marriage, a man will sell steers from his wife's herd and replace them with cows, so that in time the husband's herd shrinks as his wife's grows. At the death of the wife, her children will inherit the 'siphoned off' cattle. It appears that there are several ways of side-stepping the 'rules', and many Herero told us that they decide who inherits their wealth when they die.

Most women marry at some point in their lives, but those who were unmarried expressed ambiguity about the matter. Many women told us that marriage is preferable to the single life, but when questioned about the reasons for wanting to marry they respond with unenthusiastic Herero platitudes such as 'life without a man is like meat without salt' or 'every woman ought to have a man sitting behind her so she can rest her elbow on his knee'. Most agreed that marriage to a good man was superior to life as a single woman but that marriage to an unpleasant man, for example to a husband who would beat his wife in public, was best avoided.[8] Women's reasons for wanting to marry may be strongly motivated by economic gain.

---

[8]We never saw a man beating a woman nor did we ever see a woman with wounds. We heard one loud argument that others later called 'beating'.

In the course of our ageing study, we asked women what would make their life better. The most common answer was, 'to marry a rich man'.

Men must marry to be successful and to be regarded as proper adults. An adult male's social role is defined by *his* homestead, and this homestead must be maintained. Maintenance includes keeping the huts in good repair, cleaning the yard, and processing the milk and other domestic products. Without a wife or wives it is not possible to fulfill the adult male role.

Young men engaged to be married often spoke to us enthusiastically about their plans and about their brides-to-be. Young women would acknowledge their engagements without enthusiasm when asked and never seemed particularly interested in the topic.

Summary

The Herero were probably among the group of Bantu arriving in Southern Africa late in the last millennium BC. Unlike most of the Bantu speakers in this region, the Herero abandoned horticulture and took up pastoralism full-time. By the sixteenth century, they had moved into northern Namibia, where they have grazed cattle for hundreds of years. Genetic data and the Herero's own view of their history support the interpretation that they have been an isolated population for centuries. We believe that the apparent isolation of Herero and their neighbours has been abetted by small population sizes in this region.

Most of the ancestors of Herero came to Botswana at the turn of the century as destitute refugees. Today they are highly successful cattle pastoralists in the northern Kalahari of Botswana. Although they are enthusiastic participants in the economic and educational systems of Botswana, they retain a strong sense of ethnicity and cling to the traditions of their forefathers.

The everyday lives and the viewpoints of the two sexes seem very different in Herero society. It is interesting to compare them with the perspective of a biologist interested in comparative social and reproductive strategies. While we do not believe that this evolutionary perspective provides as much understanding as it ought to at this stage of its development, it does give us a quasi-comparative way to describe and evaluate beliefs and behaviours across cultures.

Herero women talk about social relationships as if they were sociobiologists. 'Blood' and genetic kinship are central to their descriptions of their rights in and obligations to other people. Several women told us that our European system of inheritance in which the surviving spouse would by default own the property of a dead person was unsound. After all, they reasoned, the spouse was not a relative. The property of the deceased should stay in his or her family rather than be transferred to the family of the survivor.

On the other hand this frankly biological view of social relationships did not extend to their own everyday behaviours. In this hot desert where temperatures regularly exceed 40°C they are crippled with upwards of 5 kg of gaudy Victorian dress and petticoats as well as the elaborate bonnet with 'horns' (Fig. 1.12). (A pre-adolescent girl does not wear a bonnet and is called an *otjikauhungu*, literally a 'thing with no horns'.) Their movements are slow, measured, always dignified, like those of cattle. During dances the women bob and weave so that the points of their bonnets simulate the horns of a herd. Even the custom of removing the lower incisors must be related in some way to the absence of lower incisors in cattle (J. Kurland, personal communication.) All these aspects of daily life seem scarcely related to fundamental subsistence activities like producing food or getting firewood and water. If we were inclined to interpret the 'meaning' of all this we would say that they are doing their best to be like colourful cattle.

While the everyday actions of women seem 'cultural' and their statements 'biological', the two are reversed in Herero men. Men are interested in their patrilineages (*otuzo*), their holy fires, and in the rituals and the paraphernalia associated with them. They want to have lots of children and dependents but they are explicitly not very interested in genetic relationship nor biological paternity. Several old men told us that it was proper Herero custom for old men to have a number of wives, but that boyfriends entered the huts of these wives at night since the husband was too feeble. What was important, they claimed, was the social fatherhood and *oruzo* membership of the offspring of the wives.

In contrast to the women, the men are not decorated in any obvious way. In the dry season they are up at first light and off to the wells where they work hard at watering cattle. At other times of the year they are occupied with other tasks associated with cattle management and marketing, ploughing, and tending fields in some areas, and the maintenance and manufacture of tack and other homestead equipment. When predators like lions appear they hunt them at substantial personal risk. They are soft-spoken, relaxed, and they do not express any of the complex of machismo and male posturing that is found in many societies. Their daily activities seem entirely 'biological' rather than 'cultural'.

We frankly don't know what to make of all this. An anthropologist or biologist who visited the Herero, talked to the women, and watched the men would describe people who worked hard to produce food and cattle for the market and who were interested in ecological goals and fitness in the biological sense of the term.

But an anthropologist or biologist who talked to the men and watched the women would describe people who dressed completely inappropriately for the climate to the extent of crippling themselves. Their interests and

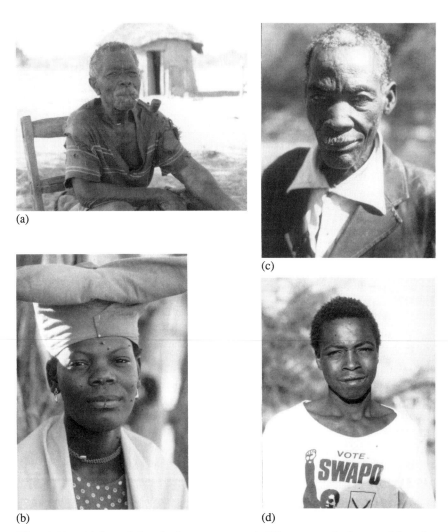

Fig. 1.12. Male and female dress contrasted. Women routinely wear Victorian dress, (b), while men dress informally, (a) and (d), except on special occassions, (c).

concerns would revolve around ritual and important cultural symbols and symbolic kinship. Ecological principles would explain little or nothing of people's activities, while seemingly autonomous and arbitrary belief systems would define the framework of daily life.

2
Field-work and methods

Introduction

The collection of good data is not a well studied aspect of demography. Since the quality and nature of data affect the scope of their usefulness and determine the validity of any conclusions drawn from them, we discuss in detail how we collected our data and how our methods may lead to various sources of bias. We also compare anthropological data collection techniques with those standard in demography. While the methods differ in scale and detail, there are big advantages in terms of data quality in smaller studies. We also discuss features of the Herero population by examining peculiarities in their age–sex pyramid.

Study area

Our study is based on interviews that we conducted in north-western Botswana between June 1987 and March 1989. Our research was carried out in several communities scattered throughout north-western Botswana (see map in Fig. 1.2). We concentrated on Herero living in the Qangwa, Nxau Nxau, Xaudum, and Xai Xai valleys; in Sehitwa and along the ridge between Bodibeng and Tsoku south-east of Sehitwa; and between Tsau and Nokaneng on the western edge of the Okavango Delta.[1] Most of the homesteads in these areas were visited at least once. We also visited a few homesteads in Thololamoro, a large settlement about 15 km north-east of Sehitwa, and in Ghanzi, a township about 200 km south-west of Sehitwa in Ghanzi district.

In 1989, the only paved road in the study area was a 120 km stretch connecting Sehitwa and Nokaneng. Because of heavy mud during the rainy season and deep sand and thick bush year-round, most of Ngamiland is accessible only by vehicles with four-wheel drive.

Maun, the district centre of Ngamiland, is only slightly more accessible. Only two decades ago Maun was a dusty village with little to offer. Today it is the outpost for tourists going on safari in the Okavango or to the Moremi and Chobe game reserves on the east side of the delta. Along with livestock ranching and diamond mining, tourism is a major industry

---

[1]These places names have been spelled many ways in the published literature. We have used the spellings typically found on maps available in Botswana.

in Botswana. Although Maun has lost its former quaintness, development of the area has probably improved the quality of life for its indigenous people. The establishment of businesses catering to tourists and safari and hunting companies also means that goods and services have become regularly available to local people. Still, there are no paved roads leading to Maun so that in many respects it remains isolated. Herero visiting Maun interact regularly with tourists but only rarely at their homesteads. Many young children we met in remote areas were afraid of us because of our unfamiliar white skin.

The climate of this region is marked by extremes. Ambient temperatures may exceed 35°C in the warm months of the year (Central Statistics Office 1988), while in the winter months it becomes cold enough at night to freeze standing water. The annual rains usually begin some time between October and December and taper off in March. It is not unusual for the rains to fail in any given year or for little or no rain to fall for many years in a row. Levels of precipitation also vary widely across narrow geographic ranges such that areas separated by only a few kilometres may receive significantly different amounts of rain in any year. The driest part of Ngamiland receives on the average 400 mm per year (Central Statistics Office 1988).

Throughout the Kalahari, rainfall is higher than in 'true' deserts, but the tendency for evaporation to exceed precipitation over the year produces an arid, desert-like environment. Consequently, Botswana is not plagued with the many diseases prevalent in the moist tropics.

The surface geology of north-western Botswana is mostly sand over porous dolomite and limestone, so that much of the rainfall is lost to the soil. The predominant vegetation of Botswana is tree savannah. The Herero habitat is dominated by scrub trees, although there are tall deciduous trees in the extreme north-west. The area is quite flat. Following the rains, grass quickly sprouts so that the Kalahari is prime cattle country. Except in the Okavango flood plain, agriculture is unreliable without irrigation. The delta swells annually during the dry season in Botswana after water from the rains in Angola flood the Okavango River, even in years of extreme drought in Ngamiland. The Okavango feeds a complex river system throughout the country. In some years, it reaches Lake Ngami, although it is usually dry. Because of shifting geologic faults, the lake does not match the glory described by travellers such as Charles Andersson (1987) who saw it in the nineteenth century.

Because of its harsh climate and scarcity of permanent water, much of Ngamiland is uninhabited. Population density of the Lake Ngami area ranges from 1 to 10 persons/km^2, but it is less than 0.1 persons/km^2 in the occupied north-western valleys and near zero in other areas west of the delta and south of Xai Xai (Central Statistics Office 1988).

Our method of sampling was to visit Herero homesteads scattered throughout the study area and to interview as many of the residents and visitors there as possible. We visited most known homesteads in the areas north of Xai Xai and the Qangwa valley at least once. Because of the higher concentration of Herero living along the Okavango Delta, a smaller proportion of the population was sampled in the Lake Ngami area. In particular, Herero living north-west of Sehitwa but south of Tsau (around Makakung) are probably under-represented. On the other hand, we interviewed individuals from these areas if we met them while interviewing Herero in other villages. We encountered large numbers of visitors in Sehitwa, Nokaneng, and Tsau, where there are medical clinics, schools, and stores. We also ascertained many individuals living in these areas indirectly through their parents and children.

We classified as Herero individuals who identified themselves as ethnically Herero. Being Herero means speaking the Herero language and following Herero customs.[2] Most of the people we interviewed were descended from either two Herero proper or two Mbanderu parents. Most of the others had mothers who were Herero proper or Mbanderu or who were adopted into either tribe as small children. Very few Herero marry outside their ethnic group. The progeny resulting from exogamous marriages, especially between Herero men and Khoisan women, were often not accepted by the Herero community.

The exact number of Herero living in our study area is unknown, but there are probably 10 000–15 000 Herero in Botswana, most of whom live in Ngamiland. In 1946, when the government of Botswana still enumerated its population by ethnic group, there were about 6000 Herero (Research Publications 1973). In Chapter 10 we project the Herero population using our estimates of demographic rates and an age structure inferred from older censuses. Our projection shows that the rate of population growth among Herero has been low until the last four decades. If there were 6000 Herero in Botswana in 1946, our calculations suggest that there were 9500 in 1986. We believe that the 1946 census under-estimated the population and that there were about 12 500 Herero in Botswana in 1986. We ascertained about 3500 individuals, and fewer than 10 per cent of them were from outside Ngamiland.

Participation in our study was voluntary, yet we received virtually 100 per cent co-operation. The few individuals who refused were either ill or busy the day we visited but offered to be interviewed another day. Occasionally, visitors who lived at neigbouring homesteads asked that we interview them at their own homestead instead. Our presence aroused interest

---

[2]Herero call their language and customs *Otjiherero*. They call themselves the *Ovaherero* (sing. *Omuherero*) and *Ovambanderu* (sing. *Omumbanderu*).

and curiosity so that interviews frequently turned into neigbourhood social gatherings while people waited around for their turn to talk with us. However, we were not always able to interview all the adults who 'belonged' to a homestead despite repeated visits because of the mobility of the population. Not only would people jump on the backs of their donkeys at the spur of the moment to visit a relative in a distant village, but they often visited for several months at a time. We knew of several people who were never home throughout the period of our study. During separate visits to the same homestead, it was possible to find a completely different group of people there each time. We also missed people who happened to be away on business (i.e. people who had gone shopping or on a cattle drive that day). Given the wide range of contexts in which we ascertained people, it is reasonable to assume that the people we interviewed were a random sample and representative of the Herero of Ngamiland.

Sampling the population

There are several ways to obtain a sample of individuals who will enter a demographic compilation. The most familiar technique is a census, an enumeration at a single time of everyone living in a defined area. Another technique often used by anthropologists is that of a family survey or register, in which individuals are ascertained when they are encountered. We used a family survey technique for several reasons, both theoretical and practical. This choice means that the appropriate statistical manipulations for our data may be different from those appropriate for the analysis of orthodox census material.

An ideal census provides a snapshot of some well-defined population at a well-defined time. In practice, of course, the snapshot is blurred—the census of Botswana, for example, extended over several weeks. For anthropologists studying a restricted area, there are some difficulties with census data. First, doing a census is a poor way to enter a new community. Many of the questions are either rude or else not quite appropriate, such as, 'Who slept here last night?' Even more mundane questions such as, 'Who owns this hut?' may be uncomfortable, as with the hut of someone recently deceased.

Second, censuses provide very little information about families. Among the Herero, individuals are very mobile. It was not uncommon to find all the *de jure* residents of homesteads away when we visited, nor was it uncommon to find that over half the people who were in a homestead were visitors whose *de jure* residences were elsewhere. Gibson (1956) describes Herero funeral visiting, for example, in which relatives of the deceased may spend many months at the wake. People looking after school-age children may live during the school term in town, and those looking after chronically ill relatives may live, temporarily, near a clinic or hospital. We encountered a few women who built huts themselves to stay in over the course of their extended visits.

Third, residence is intrinsically ambiguous. Many adults have huts in widely separated villages and they move among them over the course of a year. The mobility of children and young people is even greater. Children would show up in our neigbourhood, stay for three or four months, then go to stay with another relative. Not only did we obtain equivocal answers to queries about where such a child lived, there was in fact no single answer.

Fourth, census data are rarely collected by people with an academic interest in the data and a commitment to their quality. In many countries census takers are local government employees like teachers. Our own experiences with surrogate interviewers leads us to view with misgivings census data and census-like data (e.g. the World Fertility Survey and the Demographic and Health Surveys) collected in rural Africa. In a recent review of world-wide sex differentials in mortality, Waldron (1987) compared mortality rates from the World Fertility Survey and from 17 of the censuses that were considered most reliable by the United Nations. The correlation between the sex ratios of infant mortality rates in these two high quality data sources about the same countries at the same time was only 0.52.

We interviewed Herero in their own language (*Otjiherero*) or in !Kung (Harpending), the lingua franca of north-western Ngamiland, relying on local interpreters when necessary. We believe that our interest in learning local customs and language helped convey the importance of our work to Herero so that people we interviewed were more interested in answering our questions correctly. Because we recorded the answers ourselves, we were able to spot and correct inconsistencies and implausible answers at the time instead of having to add corrections later in our analyses. We had laptop computers with us, driven by solar panels, and we entered our information into databases every few days. This allowed us to cross-check information and to return to our informants when there were discrepancies.

Orthodox demography is based on large samples of questionnaires administered by surrogate interviewers. Administration of large data collection projects is difficult and there is little or no opportunity for interactive refinement of the questions or of the style of interviewing. Because the information that these projects collect is often of poor quality there is a large body of 'indirect techniques' for estimating vital rates. For example, demographers often use the percentage of individuals at each age whose parents are deceased to estimate adult mortality. A widespread problem with such methods is that people conducting the interviews are not careful to distinguish between biological and social parents, such as foster parents. Throughout Africa, substantial numbers of children are given to others to be reared. When asked to provide demographic information about parents, fostered children may reply about their foster parents rather than about their biological parents, especially if the biological parents are deceased (United Nations 1983; Palloni *et al.* 1984; Timæus 1986; Timæus 1991). Foster parents are typically a generation older than biological parents (see Chapter 8), so that inference about adult mortality from orphanhood can be badly biased.

We learned to frame our questions about parents specifically about 'the mother (or father) who gave birth to you'. In addition, because we collected family histories that were cross-checked every few days and because early cross-checks revealed the foster parent problem, we were able accommodate this and the cultural and linguistic problems that plague conventional demographic data collection.

Census questionnaires must by their nature be brief, so the questions that are asked are those of relevance to governments or to whomever is paying for the census. While governments are interested in the future, projecting the demand for schools, health care, etc., anthropologists are more likely to be interested in the past, in questions about group history, in culture change, and in the interaction between population and social variables over time.

Our sample was obtained by a family survey system using a method similar to the one described by Howell (1979). We interviewed as many adults as we could that we encountered, preferring women when time was short, and we entered their offspring, their parents and grandparents, their spouses, and their siblings into our database. This system has several advantages and disadvantages.

An ongoing survey and register is a polite way to obtain a set of data. Information is obtained by personal interviews with people who are well acquainted with the nature of the study. There was ordinarily a group present who would help, and several people would contribute information. Since we asked about parents and offspring, we obtained information on families, including many people not present at the interview. Children away at school, spouses away visiting or on business, and children who had been fostered elsewhere were all included. We collected systematic data on children who were fostered into the homesteads where we worked, and these children had often been ascertained through interviews with their parents elsewhere.

A difficulty with the register system among the Herero is that people are known by different names in different contexts. Most people had at least three names by which they were known, a formal Herero name, a Herero nickname, and a European name. Although most names are unique, there was always a danger that someone would be entered more than once. Herero are reluctant to speak the name of deceased loved ones so we sometimes had trouble obtaining names of parents. We recorded names of living siblings of informants so that we could match parents and guard against the problem of entering the same parent into our database under different names. In practice, weeding out duplicate parents was difficult, but we found that matching by birth year, matrilineage and patrilineage reliably identified common parents of siblings.

Guarding against duplicate entries of younger people was less of a problem because of the number of ways that they could be cross-referenced.

The population pyramid generated by a family survey is biased in complex ways due to variation in the probability of being ascertained. Adults seem to have a greater chance of being included than do children. For example, old people can enter the register by being interviewed themselves or by being named by their offspring or spouses. People of middle age can be named by their parents, themselves, their spouses, or their children. These sources of bias elevate the estimated ratio of adults to children, but we also over-estimate the proportion of children since we can ascertain children through both of their parents. Children who have been fostered out were also ascertained through their foster parents. In a closed population these biases would shrink through time as everyone became ascertained by all possible paths. The Herero population of the region where we worked is not closed, but the large number of cases where individuals were named in multiple contexts gives us confidence that the pyramid from our database is not subject to much systematic error.

In addition, because we asked people to name their spouses, their offspring, and their parents, we could cross-check and ascertain the consistency of the demographic information that we received about individuals entering our database through multiple pathways. For example, we found that men reported the same number of offspring born to their wives as their wives did, and that the year of birth that men reported for their mothers matched the answer given by their sisters. We each maintained separate databases of our interviews, and we merged these later for our demographic analysis. Our confidence in the overall quality of our data is enhanced by the lack of discrepancies between the two independently collected sets of data.

What to ask

Our interviews focused on women because they knew their own reproductive histories in more detail than their husbands or boyfriends. Men tended to be reliable informants about their own children but they often did not know much about children born to their wives or girlfriends prior or subsequent to their marriages or courtships. Nearly 40% of all births occur to unmarried women (Chapter 7). We asked women about their sequence of pregnancies and the outcome of each. We initially asked the more standard census-type question 'How many children do you have?' and obtained confused and confusing answers from reluctant informants. It seemed clear to us that we were being rude. Our experience is confirmed by Mooka (1987) writing in the analytical report of the 1981 Botswana census:

Batswana[3] generally are averse to being counted especially if the purpose is just knowing their head count. If counting has to be done, the enumerator just looks around silently and arrives at a number.

And

Batswana count their flocks, cattle, farm produce, and 'things'. When an enumerator, therefore, counts people, he/she degenerates them, reduces them, to the status of 'things'.

We eventually settled on the question, 'Did you give birth?' and then asked for the details of each birth.

Altogether, we interviewed 507 women and 195 men. We were able to determine the years of birth of all the interviewed individuals and their children as well as the years of birth of many parents, spouses, siblings, and fostered in children with Herero year names described below. We obtained 611 female reproductive histories either from women directly or from men reporting about their wives, both living and dead, from mothers reporting about their teenaged and deceased daughters, and from informants reporting about siblings. We chose to ask mothers about their young daughters because the daughters were often too bashful or embarrassed to provide reliable interviews. Young women with no children were also often away at school and would have otherwise been missed by our survey. In contrast, school-aged girls with children are often at the homestead since pregnancy forces them to quit school.

There is much reluctance among Herero to speak about deceased family members, especially if the death occurred recently. Herero say it 'hurts their hearts' to speak the name of a deceased loved one. They normally do not include deceased offspring when asked about their births, but when specifically asked they count stillborn births and early pregnancy wastage ('just blood') among their dead. We distinguished between stillborn births and neonatal mortality by asking, 'Was the baby born breathing?' A few of the women we met said that they would rather not be interviewed because they did not want to speak about offspring that they had lost. A few others refused to answer questions about spouses and parents who had died. We might worry that such refusals would lead to biases in favour of high survivorship, but these individuals invariably said something such as, 'Ask my sister over there, she can tell you about the ones who died'. We would ask them about their living family members and ask others about

---

[3]The people of Botswana call themselves *Batswana* (sing. *Mutswana*).

the dead members. Responses from informants about the years of birth and death of family members were usually the result of group discussions among kinsmen sitting in on the interviews. Our method of informal interviewing probably improved the quality of our data considerably.

A technique used by some demographers is to estimate mortality using changes in the number of deaths reported between censuses (United Nations 1983). Another popular technique is to ask about deaths that have occurred in the last year. Given the greater reluctance of individuals to discuss deaths that have occurred recently than to discuss those in the more remote past, this sampling method may be the worst method to use among Herero as well as among other ethnic groups in Botswana (Tumkaya 1987). In addition, the idea of 'within the last year exactly' is not an easy idea to get across, or rather it never seemed easy to us as ethnographers. Errors in this period can generate large errors in estimated rates. If informants misunderstand the idea of 'within a year' by three months, rates are misestimated by 25 per cent. This method also under-estimates mortality when there are no relatives left to report the death. Many of these issues are documented by Blacker (1984).

Moreover, a question about the last year does not produce very much information for the time that it takes and the pain that it (potentially) causes. A reproductive history from a 50-year-old woman furnishes about 35 person years of data on her and more person years of information about the survivorship of her offspring, while a question about whether any of her children died in the last year only furnishes one person year about her and one about each of her living children.

Among the Herero, married women often return to their mothers' homesteads to give birth. After giving birth, they are in rather strict seclusion with the new-born for several months. Residents of a homestead hosting a mother regard her as a visitor, they do not name her in a census, and she is not visible in village life. We missed interviewing many of these women directly because we either did not know about them or felt it would be rude to intrude. Yet, these are precisely the women that methods relying on events in the last year need to find. Serious bias can result from pregnancy-related movement of women (Srinivasan and Muthiah 1987).

Cultural specificity and data quality

The problems and possibilities that anthropologists face are very different from those faced by demographers and social scientists working in large-scale literate societies. Demographers are familiar with census and census-like materials, often of poor quality (Brass 1975). They are very concerned with biases, but hardly ever concerned with problems of small samples and sampling error. Anthropologists, on the other hand, are more likely to collect data of very high quality about smaller numbers of people. We must be concerned with sampling error and, we hope, less concerned with adjusting away biases.

While our own experiences with data collection among the Herero are not generalizable to other cultures, they are of interest because of the information that they provide about Herero culture. The idiosyncrasies with which we learned to cope would be absent in a neigbouring ethnic group, in which other ambiguities and difficulties would exist. In this section we discuss some peculiarities of data collection among Herero.

Ageing people who do not know their age

A very important characteristic of Herero culture for our purposes is the system of year names. In rural Africa many people do not know their own ages. Among the Herero, names are given to individual years and almost everyone knows, at least, the name of the Herero year of his or her birth. Concordances with Gregorian years are available back to about 1830 (Vedder 1966b; Gibson 1959; Irle 1906), and, most important, a person's year of birth is a significant social attribute. People typically know the names of the years of birth of friends and family members, including parents and grandparents. They also know their age-mates since there is a kind of social bond among those born in the same year.

With this system, we are able to ascertain an exact year of birth for most people in our database. There are, however, several sources of error. First, the traditional year (*ombura*, 'rain') begins in November or December when the rainy season starts, so that people who were born in, say, December 1930 may be assigned in our records to 1931 if they reported their birth year to us with a Herero year name. Second, there is some reuse of year names. There are two years of the locusts (*ojozombahu*), one in 1917 and one in 1924. When this name appeared in an interview we tried to resolve the ambiguity. We are not certain that we were always successful. In the published lists of nineteenth century names (Vedder 1966b) there are disagreements of several years for some sequences. We did not encounter any such ambiguities in the twentieth century names, but the Herero proper and the Mbanderu maintain separate names for many of the years. A set of Mbanderu year names from 1904 onwards is given in Almagor (1980). We compiled a list of year names from Vedder (1966b) and Almagor to date the years of vital events reported to us as a Herero or Mbanderu year name. This list was supplemented by year names provided by many individuals in Botswana, but especially by Titus Tjirongo, the headman of Qangwa. Our compiled list is given at the end of this chapter.

The list includes a few well-known historical events that were used to reference vital events. Usiel Kandapeaera of Thololamoro also provided us with a number of year names that are not included on this list. We were told that the year names are officially maintained by Mavazapi Tjinae of Nokaneng and Musarua Rukata of Makakung. Most Herero born after about 1960 reported events in Gregorian years.

The method of dating vital events using year names is advantageous because it is not susceptible to common problems of age estimation found in many populations, such as age-heaping on multiples of five (Brass 1968). While there is no possibility of 'digit preference' using the Herero system, there is the possibility of other kinds of bias. For example there might be prestige associated with being born in a particular year. However, few know the correspondence between the Herero year names and ages so the potential for age exaggeration is very small. People did tend to know the relative ranking of years near their own birth year since relative age is an important social attribute among the Herero. A man born in *ombura ojomapuku* probably did not know that he was born in 1928, but he probably did know that he was a year older than a friend born in *ombura ojozondendu*, 1929. We looked hard for year preferences and for discrepancies between relative ages of people and their stated birth years, and we never found evidence of either.

The !Kung Bushmen who live in north-west Ngamiland are the subject of what is perhaps the most important study ever of anthropological demography, by Nancy Howell (Howell 1979). She spent many hours tediously ranking the !Kung by age, but there were few reliable anchors to map this ranking to real years. Consequently her inferences had to be based on an assumption that the !Kung age distribution was close to that of a model stable population. In other words, it was not possible to ascertain that a certain old !Kung in her ranking was, say, 70 years old. Instead she assumed that the relative proportions of 60-, 70- and 80-year-olds were the same as those in the best fitting model life table from the Coale and Demeny (1983) tabulation. Hindsight is painfully clear—if Howell and the other members of the Harvard Kalahari Project in the 1960s (including Harpending) had explored the matter with the Herero it would have been possible to obtain exact ages of many of the !Kung since the two ethnic groups each recognize age-mates in the other group.

Other aspects of demographic interviewing

In the first week of serious data collection, after we had entered the material into our microcomputers, we discovered that the father of our interpreter had died 10 years before our interpreter was born. Thinking that we had made a recording error we checked with him. He said no, there was no mistake, his father had indeed died many years before his own birth. Why, he wondered, were we acting surprised?

Among Herero a widow often returns to her own family after the death of her husband, but she may remain with the family of her deceased husband and continue to give birth in the name of the dead husband. Our interpreter's mother had given birth to a number of children after widow-hood, and these children all acknowledged the same father. When we asked our interpreter who his *biological* father was he told us in a matter of fact way. There was no reluctance or inability to make the distinction between biological and social parents. From then on we phrased all our questions very specifically in biological terms: 'Who is the mother (or father) who gave birth to you?'[4] A more general question such as 'Who is your father?' might elicit the name of the biological father, the biological grandfather in the case of the child of an unmarried woman, a foster father, or any of the biological father's brothers.

In the same way, asking, 'Who are your children?' could generate a daz-zling diversity of answers—biological children, fostered in children, grand-children, children who had been purchased, by a man, even children from other tribes resident in the village on labour contracts might be listed. But when we asked, 'Who are the children to whom you have given birth?' we obtained exactly the information that we wanted in a demographic context.

While women and men could report both their living and dead offspring in reliable detail, we never obtained any good information on cause of death. Questions about cause of death seemed to make many people resentful and even hostile, and we stopped asking them quickly. Death is a highly loaded topic and all deaths are ultimately caused or at least abetted by sorcery, according to most informants. Such things are not the stuff of casual conversation with unfamiliar interviewers. Talking about the specifics of the deaths of individuals brings on powerful and very painful feelings in people. These feelings are not only unpleasant, they are socially dangerous.

We were able to obtain much information about sorcery, witchcraft and mortality, but only from old friends who knew us well and who knew that we would not repeat the specifics of their conversations to others. Here, for example, is an account (with the details doctored) of a death of a young middle-aged woman in which ancestors, rather than living people, are implicated:

Freda M. was an outgoing cheerful woman in her late thirties, the daughter of a very wealthy man living near the delta. Her father and mother had several daughters but no sons, so her father Gustav kept Freda at his homestead so that he would have custody of and authority over any male children that she might bear. She never married. Her father had also arranged for the widow of his classificatory younger brother to remain with him and he exercised authority over her several male offspring. Gustav was well liked and respected in the community, but he did not maintain a holy fire and was occasionally criticized for not honoring Herero traditions.

---

[4]Obviously fathers do not give birth, but this is our best translation and gets the point across.

Freda had dreams in which the ancestors warned her of her father's negligence, and she reported these, but no action was taken. Finally, she fell from a ledge and died suddenly, leaving several small children orphaned. This was taken to be a strong warning from the ancestors that traditions had to be obeyed. Gustav kindled a holy fire in his homestead and proper rituals were reinstated.

Freda had suffered from epilepsy and had had occasional seizures. Almost certainly her tragic death was brought on by a seizure while she was negotiating slippery rocks during the rainy season. But even the epilepsy was seen in retrospect as part of the scheme of the ancestors to express their disapproval of the neglect of traditional ways in Gustav's village.

The custody of one small child of Freda's was given by the family to her mother, a vigorous woman in her early sixties. Another was given to Freda's sister. Several months after the death, senior family members of the (biological) father of Freda's oldest daughters arrived to request that their family be allowed to purchase genetricial rights in these daughters. One of these daughters was already married and the other was engaged. After several weeks of negotiation, payment was arranged and custody was transferred. The fee was two cows for the daughters and two cows as a seduction fee.

Freda was a friend of ours, and we know about her epilepsy because we discussed it with her in 1987. After her death this prior neurological problem was hardly mentioned nor even acknowledged. The point is that we would not have obtained the information in a retrospective interview, and we would have aroused strong feelings of guilt and danger by pursuing the precise circumstances of the death.

A few people agreed with our own assessment that witchcraft was superstition. These non-believers were agnostics rather than followers of a competing belief system. Among the more spiritually inclined Herero, the ancestor cult, Protestant Christianity, vigilance, and the struggle against witchcraft were part of an apparently harmonious system of beliefs and practices. There was often debate, for example, about the relative efficacy of traditional and Christian practitioners for combating the onslaught of sorcery from others.

The age–sex distribution

Fig. 2.1 shows the age–sex distribution of 2591 individuals in our database by single years. This pyramid reflects the age–sex structure of the living Herero population in 1986. Such a display is not very useful since the differences from year to year are great and the overall impression is one of random noise with little pattern. The jaggedness reflects both signal and noise-signal in the sense that the shape reflects epidemics and droughts and other events in history that changed the risk of death of people, especially of children, and noise in the sense that the numbers in any single age–sex category are small and subject to much statistical fluctuation.

The structure of an African pastoralist community

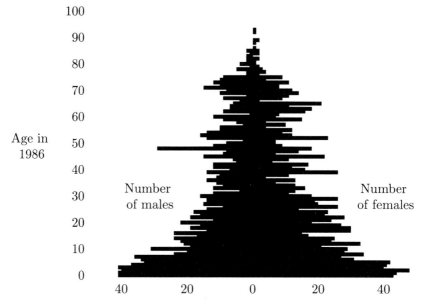

Fig. 2.1. Age–sex pyramid of living Herero in 1986 by single year.

A traditional approach to coping with the noise is to collapse the counts into 5-year intervals as in Fig. 2.2. Properties of these pyramids are well summarized in Young (1971) or any demography textbook. Broad based pyramids are produced by high fertility populations, while low fertility populations have narrow-based pyramids. Narrow-based pyramids are also found in populations with very high mortality. Qualitatively, the Herero pyramid is narrow like that of a low fertility population, especially for people older than 20. It is more like the pyramid of an eastern European country with a shrinking population than like the pyramid of a typical African country with a high birth-rate. At the base of the pyramid, there is broadening, suggesting increased fertility in recent decades. There are some asymmetries between the sexes, especially in the older age groups, but it is difficult to evaluate the significance of these because of the limited sample size.

Smoothing data

The tradition of lumping people into 5-year categories is well established, but it is a hold-over from the days when computers were distant and difficult resources. Today, it is an abuse of good data. Collapsing the series into 5-year age groups amounts to computing 5-year running averages, then discarding four of the five data points from the result. Anthropologists must

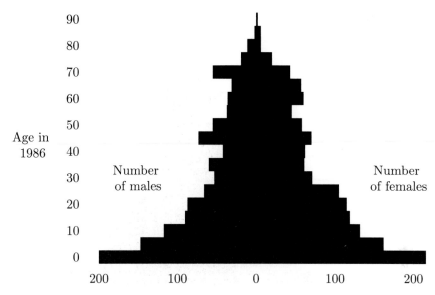

Fig. 2.2.   Age–sex pyramid of living Herero in 1986 by 5-year age groups.

struggle with extracting as much information as possible from small samples, and a more sophisticated approach to examining the age–sex structure is desirable. Fig. 2.3 shows the raw counts smoothed by computing a seven-point tapered moving average of the raw age counts—the number of individuals of each age is replaced by a weighted mean of the numbers in neigbouring age groups.

Filter construction is a mixture of common sense and black art. For example, a recent review of smoothing techniques (Goodall 1990) repeats a recommendation (Silverman 1986) that a series be smoothed until it looks about right but has 'a few additional wiggles ... to think about'. We have experimented with various filters applied to the data in Fig. 2.1, and we always obtain something like Fig. 2.3. Since the purpose of smoothing is exploratory rather than confirmatory, it is probably not of much consequence which one we present. The algorithm that we use has the advantage of being simple.

Details of the age structure

It appears that the dramatic tragedy of the 1904 war still echoes in the Herero age pyramid. There seems to be a wave in the population of 22–25-year duration. There are birth surges peaking among the population aged in their early 20s, middle 40s, and middle 60s. Troughs occur at the ages of 15, 35, and 60. Censuses taken in the 1950s by Gibson (1959) and

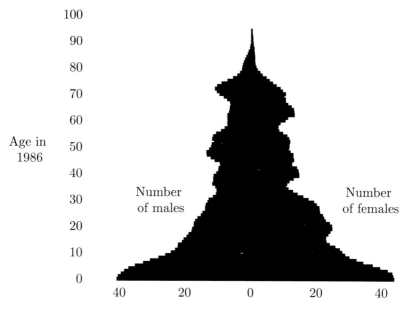

Fig. 2.3. Age–sex pyramid of living Herero in 1986 by single year, smoothed by a tapered moving average.

Günther Wagner (Köhler 1959 *a*; Köhler 1959 *c*; Köhler 1959 *b*; Köhler 1959 *d*; Wagner 1957) show that there was a disproportionate number of females below age 20 among the survivors of the 1904 massacre. This bulge of females still echoes in the pyramid today. In Chapter 10 we project this immigrant population from 1904 to the present using reconstructed age-specific fertility and mortality rates, and we obtain a pyramid with the same wave and shape as Fig. 2.3.

The implied generation time in this wave seems too short. Most human populations have generation times of 25–30 years, about 6 years longer than the apparent wave in Fig. 2.3. But the Herero have suffered from pathological sterility that terminated the reproductive careers of many women early in their twenties leading to a shortened generation time. The natural period of the Leslie matrix constructed from the fertility rates of the first half of this century is in fact 22 years (Chapter 10).

The male pyramid shows the same general pattern as that of the females, except that the bulge of individuals born in the 1960s is missing. The missing bulge on the male side suggests either that there was a particularly marked aberration in the secondary sex ratio in the sixties, or that males have experienced much higher levels of infant and childhood mortality than have females. We see in the next chapter that the second suggestion is supported by our data.

List of Herero and Mbanderu year names

These are compiled from Almagor (1980), Vedder (1966*b*), and the note-book of Titus Tjirongo, the Qangwa headman. A number of Herero we met in Botswana contributed additional events and year names.

1832 *ojongombe ombonde*
1833 *ojomeva*
1834 *ojozombahe*
1835 *ojondaambe*
1836 *ojondjouojakaveta*
1837 *ojetemba*
1838 *ojorokue*
1839 *ojekuva*
1840 *ojorukoro*
1841 *ojohara*
1842 *ojongungu*
1843 *ojondukua*
1844 *ojokaambi*
1845 *ojorupera*
1846 *ojomandjembere*
1847 *ojonganga*
1848 *ojorukata*
1849 *ojohange*
1850 *ojodjindjumba*
1851 *ojozondema*
1852 *ojovihende*
1853 *ojondjuuojarukoro*
1854 *ojomevaomengi*
1855 *ojumbua*
1856 *ojorukamburo*
1857 *ojondorozo*
1858
1859 *ojunganiua*
1860 *ojombondi*
1861 *ojondujundiuo*
1862 *ojepunga*
1863 *ojotjikesatjazeraua*
1864 *ojongangajambaka*
1865 *ojotjikoruha*
1866 *ojorupati*
1867 *ojerambo*

1868 *ojongombeongange*
1869 *ojomukaaru*
1870 *ojoheo*
1871 *ojotungava*
1872 *ojesuru*
1873 *ojomatupa*
1874 *ojotjinenge (ojotjimenga?)*
1875 *ojomuambo*
1876 *ojerunga*
1877 *ojohaka (ojohara?)*
1878 *ojourombo*
1879 *ojeraka*
1880 *ojongombeonganga*
1881 *ojomativa*
1882 *ojohava*
1883 *ojongoze*
1884 *ojonjose*
1885 *ojovitenda*
1886 *ojotjioua tjakurukuii*
1887 *ojorundumba*
1888 *ojondimbu*
1889 *ojondjeo*
1890 *ojongamero o tjipuka*
1891 *ojozembahu*
1892 *ojondjuo*
1893 *ojondjenge*
1894 *ojondorozu*
1895 *ojongue ja karoui*
1896 *ojozehungu*
1897 *opesa*
1898 *ojotjindjumba*
1899 *ojoruara*
1900 *ojondembonde*
1901 *ojongose*
1902 *ojomueze*
1903 *ojogarangombe*
1904 *ojondjembo, ojondjembo jo vaherero*
1905 *ojoruvara, ojonjota*
1906 *ojotjikoroha*
1907 *ojorutjindo, ojakorusuvero*
1908 *ojomunguindi,* (Sekgoma goes to Kavimba), *ojomunguendi*
1909 *ojozonde*
1910 *ojomapuku*

1911 *ojomuukuani, ojomuhana*
1912 *ojorutjindo, ojorutjindo ra Sekgoma*
1913 *ojoviposa, ojongombosazu, ojongombeosazu*
1914 *ojombongarero, ojondjembo,* (birth of Kakaha), *ojotjitundu*
1915 *ojondjembo, ojovitoto*
1916 *ojokaumbo, ojokaurumbo*
1917 *ojozombahu, ojotjihenga*
1918 *ojorutjindo, ojotjikoroha*
1919 *ojombepo*
1920 *ojoikambe, ojoukombe*
1921 *ojakaupaha*
1922 *ojozongamero, ojoseemana*
1923 *ojotjikesa, ojotjikesa tja Samuel na Khama*
1924 *ojozombahu, ojozombahu ozondenga*
1925 *ojomevomengi, ojoue jakambo*
1926 *ojokatuahuurua,* (Nicodemus from Kavimba to Rakops), *ojongameero*
1927 *ojeteva*
1928 *ojomapuku, ojorura, ojotungava*
1929 *ojozondendu*
1930 *ojovitoro, ojokarumburumbu*
1931 *ojomueze, ojondimbu jakamburee, ojotii*
1932 *ojondu, ojomevauasevitura, ojondondimbu*
1933 *ojokainahange, ojozohorongo*
1934 *ojoenda, ojotii*
1935 *ojorutjindo, ojomuukuani*
1936 ? (a fruit), *ojozombua*
1937 *ojokuhavera, ojomoremi III ndjohavero ko tjihavero*
1938 *ojondorongo, ojondorongo jo mepane*
1939 *ojomarongerero, ojovahona*
1940 *ojorutjindo, ojoserandu*
1941 *ojovanatje, ojovita ua Hitral*
1942 *ojahuriua*
1943 *ojondiro,* (epidemic kills calves in Sehitwa), *ojombaova*
1944 *ojombuise,* (people began dying of plague in Sehitwa), *ojaruzize, ojomevomengi*
1945 *ojondirojomuhona, ojozomburu*
1946 *ojomeero,* (end of Sehitwa plague), *ndjata moreme, ojomasole tjivakotoka*
1947 *ojotjikesa, ojozomidiva ozengi*
1948 *ojondjembomehi, ojondjara, ojoleuba*
1949 *ojotjihamunika*
1950 *ojourumbu*
1951 *ojonjati*

1952 *ojomeero*
1953 *ojondiro, ojehi tjira njenga njenga*
1954 *ojomamutao*
1955 *ojaeliezer*
1956 *ojozohima*
1957 *ojomaahero, ojozongombe za Tsumkwe, ojozongombe za tjizakahua*
1958 *ojozondjo*
1959 *ojokapara, ojondiro ja Tshekedi Khama*
1960 *ojoviposa*
1961 *ojomeero*
1962 *ojondorongo*
1963 *ojourunga*
1964 *ojondjombo*
1965 *ojorambu*
1966 *ojomauaneno*
1967 *ojotjiposa*
1968 *ojouenda*
1969 *ojondiro*
1970 *ojokaitukire*
1971 *ojomueze*
1972 *ojoviposa*
1973 *ojondiro*
1974 *ojozonde, lethobo, ojorutobo*
1975 *ojorutjindo*
1976 *ojakomihoko*
1977 *ojerakanotjikoti*
1978 *ojomaazemeno*
1979
1980 *ojondiro jatautona S. Khama*
1981 *ojondiro jo Muhona Letsholathebe*
1982 *ojondiro ja Lenjeletse*
1983
1984
1985
1986 *ojonjose*

3
Infant and childhood mortality

Introduction

In this chapter we discuss levels and trends in infant and childhood mortality. Early mortality is a standard indicator of the overall health of a population, so we are interested in comparing Herero rates at different periods and with infant and childhood mortality in other populations. In particular the !Kung Bushmen, the subjects of Nancy Howell's (1979) pioneering demographic study, inhabit the same area and should be exposed to similar pathogens. The !Kung have less food than the Herero and they are thinner. A comparison between the two groups may show the effects of diet on early mortality.

We are also interested in the sex ratio of mortality. This is a lively topic in both demography and anthropology although the two disciplines have rather different perspectives on the matter. While male preference has been widely reported and analysed, the Herero show the other pattern—female survival through infancy and childhood greatly exceeds that of males. In this chapter we describe overall mortality and attempt to model the female preference. In Chapter 9 we compare Herero mortality patterns with those of their !Kung Bushmen neigbours.

Sex preference

Demographers are interested in the social and economic determinants of the widespread excess mortality of females that is especially pronounced in south Asia (Waldron 1987; Muhuri and Preston 1991; Freed and Freed 1989; Miller 1981; Miller 1984). The evidence from south Asia is of two sorts, censuses that show a shortage of females and direct demographic tabulations of infant and childhood mortality by sex. These tabulations (e.g. D'Souza and Chen 1980; Simmons *et al.* 1982) reveal a hazard ratio in favour of males of about 1.5, that is to say girls are approximately half again as likely to die in infancy or childhood as boys. Distal determinants of the mortality differential seem to be the expense of dowries in these intensive agricultural societies and the utility of male but not female offspring for providing agricultural labour. Proximate determinants are discriminatory feeding practices and more diligent provision of medical care to males.

An excellent treatment of the social context of this kind of sex bias is given by Dickemann (1979). She describes these as 'hypergynous dowry' systems in which the families of females must compete with each other to obtain (literally purchase) husbands for their daughters. They are hypergynous because there is a class or caste hierarchy and families with more money than the average for their class or caste achieve upward mobility by marrying their daughters into higher classes. At the top of the hierarchy there are excess females whose parents did not buy them into the reproductive system because of the expense and they do not reproduce, at least in the socially appropriate context. The model predicts that at the bottom of the social ladder a symmetrical preference for females and neglect of males should occur although this has not been described anywhere. Boone (1988) describes a similar mating system in medieval Portugal.

Dickemann's model of high status families' son preference was derived from a more general model of sex ratio manipulation proposed by Trivers and Willard (1973). They pointed out that if the overall condition of a mother affects the condition of her offspring and if the individual fitness of one sex in a species is more variable than that of the other, optimizing parents should bias the sex of their offspring. Mammalian mothers in good condition should produce male offspring, since the reproductive biology of mammals allows huge variance in male fitness but not so much variance in female fitness. Females in bad condition should produce daughters because the fitness of daughters is not so dependent on their condition.

Anthropologists have looked for manifestations of this effect in human societies, reasoning that wealthy or high status families should produce more sons, low status families more daughters. Evidence for strategic variation in sex ratio at birth is not compelling (Sieff 1990). Differential treatment of sons and daughters has been well documented, but it does not always follow the prediction of the Trivers and Willard model (Cronk 1991). There are few examples of bias in favour of females. One probable case of female bias among a low status group has been given by Cronk (1989) among the Mukogodo of Tanzania, people who switched from foraging to pastoralism under pressure of contact with Maasai early in this century. They favour daughters through longer lactation and more visits to clinics. There is a suggestion that female survival exceeds that of males, but the numbers are small.

Male preference in Asia has received widespread attention from demographers and anthropologists in part because it is not hidden—adults are not reticent about their preference for sons. Margery Wolf (1972, p. 54), for example, reports that in traditional Taiwan a new-born daughter with older sisters was in grave peril—'If the family had a surfeit of girls, she was simply allowed to slip into a bucket of water, and that was the end of it'.

On the other hand, indications of sex preference are conspicuously absent from African ethnographies, and, when asked, most rural Africans say that they want any children that they can have. The census of Botswana remarks on the absence of sex preference in the country (Mooka 1987). On the other hand, some published numbers suggest a different picture. In a survey of sex differential in infant mortality, Ohadike (1983) found that male infant mortality in sub-Saharan African countries often exceeds that of females by a factor of 1.5. The Botswana Family Health Survey (Lesetedi *et al.* 1989) found that male infants suffered a relative risk of infant death of 1.5 compared to females in the whole country. These demographic indicators of sex preference are as great or greater than those found in south Asia!

This brief look at the literature about sex biased treatment of infants and children suggests that there are two rather different issues that are easily confounded. One issue is whether parents systematically treat one sex better than the other. The second issue is whether parents *say that they* prefer one sex over the other. The demographic data suggest that male preferential treatment is widespread in Asia and that female preferential treatment may be widespread in sub-Saharan Africa. Anthropological evidence suggests that public articulation of preference is limited to Asia.

Chapter overview

In the rest of this chapter we discuss tabulations of infant and childhood mortality obtained from reproductive histories. These show that males have been approximately three times as likely to die in infancy as females and twice as likely to die in childhood.

We then derive a model of asymmetric helping between opposite sex siblings. Our model suggests hypotheses about patterns of mortality; we test these predictions and find only weak support for our model. Finally, we use logistic regression and a likelihood ratio test inductively to identify correlates of male and female mortality in our data and to test for heterogeneity among mothers in the survival of their children.

At the end of the chapter we describe Herero explanations of the bias and speculate further about why bias is articulated in south Asia but not in sub-Saharan Africa.

Infant and childhood mortality among Herero

Reproductive histories

Data quality

We might distrust data from reproductive histories because of the possibility that older women forget past births, especially those of dead children. We have looked for indications of this recall bias in our reproductive histories, but we find little or no evidence for it.

If older women forget births that they had many years in the past, especially those who died, tabulations of mortality should show suspiciously low rates in the distant past. We find instead that infant and childhood death rates reported by our oldest informants are consistent with those of model life tables that we calculated using estimators of adult survivorship (e.g. maternal orphanhood, see Newell 1988), and older women report higher rates of infant and childhood death among their offspring than do younger women. Both infant and childhood mortality have been declining in this century. There is no indication of sex ratio distortion in the reports of older informants, as might occur if they were preferentially forgetting one sex or the other.

Another prediction of the theory that older women forget their children is that they should preferentially forget their earlier births. The age pattern of lifetime fertility obtained by recall should look too extended, too concentrated in the later years of child-bearing. Our data show the opposite pattern—fertility was concentrated early rather than late in the reproductive span of our older informants compared to the normal human pattern of age-specific fertility (see Chapter 10). These are all indications that older women are not forgetting offspring. It is difficult to believe that women actually forget births, but it is easy to believe that they have little interest in speaking casually about children that they have lost.

Results

Tables 3.1 and 3.2 show temporal trends in overall infant and childhood mortality as tabulated from reproductive histories. Both infant and childhood rates decline over time, with rates in recent cohorts about half the rates suffered by children born before 1960. Infant mortality has gone from about 130 per 1000 live births to 60, while childhood mortality has fallen from 80 per 1000 to about 30. These levels of mortality are much lower than those of !Kung Bushmen in the same region (Howell 1979; Harpending and Wandsnider 1982), and they are also lower than rates for much of the rest of rural Africa (Hill and Hill 1988). The female infant mortality rate is the same as the female rate for Botswana as a whole reported by the 1988 *Family health survey* (Lesetedi *et al.* 1989). The recent Herero male infant mortality rate, on the other hand, is double that of the whole country, 95 per 1000 vs 48.

These comparisons with national level figures should be regarded as coarse-grained only. The two Family Health Surveys of Botswana, one undertaken in 1984 (Manyeneng *et al.* 1985) and one in 1988 (Lesetedi *et al.* 1989), found infant mortality rates that differed by a factor of 1.7 *for the same time period*. Manyeneng *et al.* (1985) did not report sex differences. The overall rate was 70 per 1000 for 1977–81, in agreement with the 1981 census. The 1988 survey found a rate of 38 for 1983–8, composed of a rate of 48 per 1000 for male births and 32 for female. The latter survey found a rate of 42 for 1978–82.

Table 3.1. Infant mortality by period

	Males			Females		
	−1959	1960–1974	1975–	−1959	1960–1974	1975–
At risk	262	283	401	224	257	394
Deaths	32	45	38	30	18	12
Mortality rate	0.12	0.16	0.09	0.13	0.07	0.03

Table 3.2. Childhood (ages 1–4) mortality by period

	Males			Females		
	−1959	1960–1974	1975–	−1959	1960–1974	1975–
At risk	230	238	253	194	239	265
Deaths	24	20	10	13	9	6
Mortality rate	0.10	0.08	0.04	0.07	0.04	0.02

A similar temporal decline in mortality is found throughout Africa, but the cause is not clear (Hill and Hill 1988). Before the early 1970s there were only occasional visits by dispensers of medicine to rural areas of north-western Botswana, while recently many clinics staffed by nurses have been established. But the occasional availability of a dispenser does not seem adequate to explain the mortality decline from 1940 to 1955.

These tables also show that the mortality decline is not so straightforward when the sexes are considered separately. The drop in infant mortality is essentially a decline in the mortality of female infants. For births before the 1960s, for example, male and female infant mortality rates were similar while since the early 1960s female rates have dropped sharply and male rates have remained about the same or risen slightly during the 1960s.

These rates show strong excess mortality of males. This was suggested by the age–sex pyramid in Chapter 2 that showed an excess of females in their 20s and younger.

Table 3.3 shows the two-by-two contingency table testing for a sex difference in infant mortality in the two recent cohorts of Tables 3.1 and 3.2. The p-value for the null hypothesis of no sex difference in risk is less than 1 in 1 million. Table 3.4 is the same test for sex differences in childhood mortality. The difference is significant at a level of 1 in 100, reflecting a smaller relative risk and fewer deaths, because childhood mortality is much lower than infant mortality. We conclude that females do much better in infancy and probably childhood than do males and that this sex biased survival is recent, appearing in the 1960s with the increase in fertility and, perhaps, higher demands on young women for parental investment.

Table 3.3. Infant mortality by sex since 1960. The value of the X^2 statistic is 30.7, $p \approx 10^{-6}$. The estimated relative risk of infant mortality for males to females is 2.9

	Males	Females
Survivors	601	621
Deaths	83	30

Table 3.4. Childhood mortality by sex since 1960. The value of the X^2 statistic is 6.3, $p \approx 0.01$. The estimated relative risk of childhood mortality for males to females is 2.1

	Males	Females
Survivors	461	489
Deaths	30	15

Male mortality is often higher than that of females. In the Coale and Demeny (1983) model West series at level 15, for example, the mortality of females is about 100 per 1000, of males 120. But among Herero, male infant mortality is between two and three times that of females—a difference that is much greater than any inherent male vulnerability would induce.

Sex ratio

The numbers in Table 3.1 show that the shortage of males born in the 1960s and later is not due to any aberration in secondary sex ratio. Since 1960 there are 684 male births and 651 female births, for an estimated secondary sex ratio of 105. There is a slight excess of males, and we can conclude without tests that a statistical fluctuation in the sex ratio of live births does not account for the missing males in the population pyramid.

Indirect inference

Fig. 3.1 shows the proportion of all live births that are dead today by age of mother in our sample. The two series in the figure represent proportions of male and female offspring that are dead. The proportions of each sex who are dead today are about the same for mothers over the age of 55, while younger women have lost significantly more of their males. For comparison,

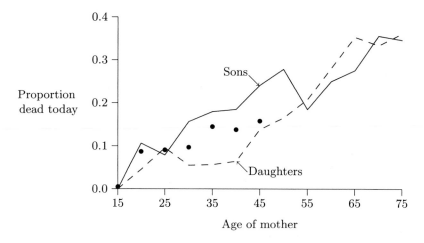

Fig. 3.1. Proportion of children dead at time of interview, by age of mother. Male and female children are shown as solid and dashed lines, while the bullets show corresponding figures with both sexes pooled from the 1984 Botswana Family Health Survey. The FHS report did not distinguish between male and female offspring.

the proportions, with sex of offspring pooled, found by the 1984 Botswana FHS are also shown in the figure.

Fig. 3.1 reveals in a different way the trends that we discussed above. First, it shows that males suffer from a greatly increased risk of mortality. Second, it shows that this sex difference in risk began in the late 1950s or early 1960s and that there is no evidence for it in earlier cohorts.

An exploratory look at the mortality drop

It is desirable to examine the pattern of change in infant mortality through time so as to understand its connections with other events in Herero history, but with small numbers there is always the danger of over-interpretation of noise. We have constructed Fig. 3.2 as an exploratory look at the details of change, but we emphasize that the look must be cautious. The lines are smoothed 10-year moving averages of male and female infant mortality rates. The point for the male rate in 1960, for example, is computed as the number of infant deaths between 1955 and 1965 divided by the number of births between 1955 and 1965. The point for 1961 is the same quotient for births between 1956 and 1966. This series was then smoothed by a Hanning filter.

Fig. 3.2 seems to show clear trends. Before the 1960s female mortality

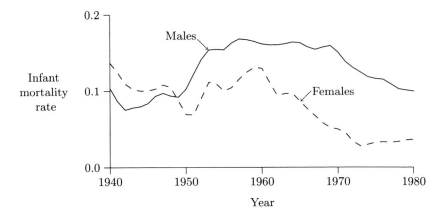

Fig. 3.2. Infant mortality rates through time. The difference between male and female rates before 1950 is based on small numbers and is not meaningful, while the difference in the 1960s and later is based on large numbers and is highly significant.

exceeded that of males, while since the 1960s male mortality has been greater than that of females. The crossover occurred in the 1950s. But smoothing of data series, like many other complex statistical techniques, always gives an answer that can be interpreted, and humans like to see pattern even when it is absent. A glance at Table 3.1 shows that the excess female mortality in the past is not based on large numbers of infant deaths and that it should not be accepted with any degree of confidence. The recent excess male mortality, on the other hand, is highly significant. The smoothing shown in Fig. 3.2 is valuable in showing how this developed, but it is only valuable when our other eye is on Table 3.1 to help differentiate solid from spurious pattern.

A model of sex preference

No informant ever suggested a preference for a child of one sex or the other to us. Sex preference is not found in Botswana as a whole (Mooka 1987), and it is conspicuously absent from most sub-Saharan African ethnography. On the other hand, from an economic viewpoint there is the idea that daughters bring in cattle to the family through their reproduction, while the reproduction of sons costs cattle. Among the Herero, bride-wealth is small, on the order of one or two cows along with cash, but there are other mechanisms through which females bring in wealth. Fathers of the children of unmarried women often purchase patrilineal rights in their children, and 'seduction fees' and 'child fees' can be much higher than bride-wealth.

This leads us to consider a model of asymmetric helping between siblings. In the Herero case, the idea is that a sister contributes to the fitness of her brother while a brother does not contribute to the fitness of his sister. This means that a daughter is more 'valuable', in the currency of fitness, than a son, especially if there are sons who will be the beneficiaries of the cattle earned by her. Our model may apply in other contexts, for example in situations of chronic raiding and warfare males may defend their sisters while receiving no fitness benefits from their sisters. Here the helping sex is males, but the formalism is the same.

We develop a Darwinian model because the formalisms and mechanisms are well understood in population genetics, although the translation to an economic model would be straightforward. Simmons *et al.* (1982) posit an economic model to account for preferential treatment of males in rural India, but their logic is similar to ours. Rogers (1990) shows that under very general conditions where fitness depends on heritable wealth, wealth is a better proxy for long term contribution to future generations than is number of offspring.

We reason from the viewpoint of a mother. Since fitnesses are relative we choose that of a daughter as a baseline so that any daughter has an expected fitness of 1. A son's expected fitness depends on the number of adult brothers and sisters that he has. Let w_0 be the expected fitness of a son with no sisters, and let the fitness of a son with d sisters and $s - 1$ brothers be

$$w_0(1 + \alpha \frac{d + d_f}{s}).$$

This model implies that the expected fitness of a son increases with the number of women who will provide cattle for him and decreases with the number of his brothers who will compete for those cattle. The term d_f ('free daughters') arises from the contribution to male fitness of women who have daughters but no sons; it is assumed that the income from these daughters is dispersed at random. The parameter α measures the contribution of a daughter to her brother's Darwinian fitness; if α is 0.1 it means that a sister adds 10 per cent to her brother's fitness.

We now assume that the distributions of sons and daughters within sibships are independent and that a fraction π of sibships contains no sons. If the average number of daughters per sibship is $\bar{d}$, then

$$d_f = \frac{\bar{d}\pi}{1 - \pi}.$$

The expected fitness of the offspring of the ith mother who has (or expects to have) s_i sons and d_i daughters is just d_i through her daughters and

$$w_0(s_i + \alpha(d_i + d_f))$$

through her sons if she has at least one; 0 if she has none.

The population totals of these sibship fitnesses are:

Sons	Daughters
$w_0(\bar{s} + (1 - \pi)\alpha(\bar{d} + d_f))$	$\bar{d}$

Since everyone has one father and one mother, the population total fitness of all sons must be equal to that of all daughters. Equating these, substituting for d_f, and solving for w_0, we obtain the value of a son with no sisters,

$$w_0 = \frac{\bar{d}}{\bar{s} + \alpha\bar{d}}$$

or in terms of the population sex ratio $r = \bar{s}/\bar{d}$

$$w_0 = \frac{1}{r + \alpha}.$$

If there is no asymmetric helping, that is if $\alpha = 0$, then the fitness of a male relative to a female is just the inverse of the sex ratio as in classical Fisherian theory.

Asymmetric helping will select for a biased sex ratio. This ratio can be found by noting that, at equilibrium, the average fitness consequence *to a parent* in the population of bearing a son must equal that of bearing a daughter. The average change in the fitness of a parent caused by the birth of a son at equilibrium is $1/(r + \alpha)$, while the change caused by the birth of a daughter is $1 + \alpha/(r + \alpha)$. Equating these, we find that the equilibrium sex ratio should be

$$\hat{r} = 1 - 2\alpha.$$

There are three implications of this model that can be compared to data from the Herero. First, since the sex ratio at birth is slightly greater than 1, females will on average be 'worth' more than males in terms of the mother's fitness. The prediction is that parental care will be better for females and their survival should be better. Unfortunately, we knew this to be true before we derived the model.

The second implication is that the excess value of females should be less when there is much infertility in the population because infertility leads to smaller families and more sibships with no males. Therefore, fertility increase should lead to a greater sex differential in survivorship. In our case, the recovery from infertility meant a change in total fertility from about 3 to about 7, and the sex differential in survival appeared as fertility increased. But we also knew this before we derived the model.

The third implication is that a previous living sibling of the opposite sex should protect a new-born. A new-born boy is more valuable, in the

Table 3.5. Logistic regression analysis of mortality in the first 2 years. The likelihood ratio X^2 statistic is 11.0 with 4 d.f., $p \approx 0.027$ for males, 28.0 with 4 d.f., $p \approx 10^{-5}$ for females

Variable	Male mortality		Female mortality	
	t-Value	Significance	t-Value	Significance
Birth-year	1.8	0.08	1.0	0.34
Prior sib deaths	−2.4	0.07	−5.3	0.00
Living sisters	1.4	0.16	3.4	0.00
Living brothers	2.3	0.02	4.1	0.00

currency of his mother's fitness, if he has a living older sister, because this sister will bring in cattle that will help him reproduce. Similarly, a new-born girl is more valuable if she has a living older brother since she contributes not only to her own fitness but also an increment to the expected fitness of her brother. Prior siblings of the same sex should have no effect, according to this model, nor should the numbers of previous siblings. Tabulating deaths in the first 2 years of life according to whether, at the time of birth, a child had a living sibling of either sex, we found that

1. A prior living sister does protect a new-born boy, as predicted, $X_1^2 = 6.9$, $p \approx 0.01$.

2. A prior living brother does not protect a new-born girl, contrary to the prediction, $X_1^2 = 0.58$, not significant.

3. A prior living sister does not protect a new-born girl, as predicted, $X_1^2 = 1.48$, not significant.

4. A prior living brother does not protect a new-born boy, as predicted, $X_1^2 = 1.7$, not significant.

We conclude that our model does not provide a very good explanation of the observed mortality patterns. But the model could be modified in many ways; for example it might incorporate competition or co-operation between members of the same sex, and these effects could be specified in many ways. With no clear direction, we undertook an exploratory logistic regression analysis of mortality in the first 2 years of life against several basic demographic variables.

Correlates of early mortality

This logistic regression is restricted to the 1221 offspring of mothers between 30 and 55 years of age because these children are the cohort that experienced the very strong sex bias. Predictor variables are year of birth, the number of living sisters of the child at the time of the child's birth, the number of living brothers, and the number of prior siblings who were dead at the time of birth. Table 3.5 shows the results of this exercise.

There are two surprising patterns. First, female mortality is much more 'predictable' than is male mortality, which seems on these grounds more random. Second, in both sexes mortality risk increases with previous dead siblings but declines with the number of previous living siblings of both sexes. The best predictor of whether a new-born of either sex will survive for 2 years is whether his or her older siblings survived. These results suggest that there is heterogeneity among mothers in their ability to keep their children alive and that the risk factors for infant and early childhood death are characteristics of the mothers rather than of the child.

Maternal heterogeneity in offspring survivorship

We constructed a likelihood ratio test of the the hypothesis that there is heterogeneity among mothers against the null hypothesis that all children share a common risk independent of who their mother is. Specifically, the null hypothesis is that the probability of death before age 2 is the same for each mother. The alternate hypothesis specifies that there are two kinds of mothers, 'good' mothers and 'bad' mothers, and that the risk of death is less for offspring of the former than it is for the latter. We fit this model separately for male and female offspring.

The one parameter null model depends on the risk of death before age 2, p. The likelihood of a mother who had $l + d$ births, l of which survived and d of which died, is then proportional to

$$p^d (1 - p)^l.$$

If a fraction π of mothers are 'good' mothers and experience a risk p_g of losing a child while a fraction $1 - \pi$ are 'bad' and experience a risk p_b, the likelihood of the same mother's experience is

$$\pi p_g^d (1 - p_g)^l \; + \; (1 - \pi) p_b^d (1 - p_b)^l.$$

The likelihood of the whole data set is the product of likelihoods of each mother, so the log-likelihood is the sum of the natural logarithms. Estimates of the parameters π, p_b, and p_g were obtained by an iterative procedure that found the maximum of the likelihood surface. Twice the difference between the log-likelihoods of the two models is approximately a χ^2 variate with two degrees of freedom under the null hypothesis that there is no heterogeneity, i.e. that p_b and p_g are the same and equal to the overall p. There are two degrees of freedom because two is the difference between three parameters of the full model and one parameter of the null model.

For daughters, the one parameter model that all women are subject to a risk of 0.06 of losing a new-born girl has a log-likelihood of -134.1.[1] The best fitting alternate model is that 72 per cent of mothers never lose a daughter while the remaining mothers experience a risk of 0.20. This alternate hypothesis has a log-likelihood of -127.1. Twice the difference between these is 13.4 with an associated p-value of 0.001 from a χ^2 table with two degrees of freedom. There is highly significant heterogeneity among Herero mothers in the survivorship of their daughters.

For sons, the one parameter model finds a risk of loss of 0.16 and a log-likelihood of -283.1. The two-class model finds that 55 per cent of the mothers experience a risk of 0.03 of losing a new-born male, while the remaining 45 per cent of mothers experience a risk of 0.30. The latter model has a log-likelihood of -273.8, twice the difference is 18.6, and the associated p-value is approximately 0.0001. Again there is significant heterogeneity among women.

The specific parameter estimates of the heterogeneous models should probably not be taken seriously since we could just as well fit models of three kinds of mothers, or four, or five, and they would give very different impressions. But the existence of heterogeneity is statistically highly significant and suggests that proximal causes of mortality should be sought in characteristics of low and high risk mothers. For evolutionary modelling the suggestion is that there is meaningful variation among mothers, perhaps in parental investment strategy or health. Characteristics of mothers should be the focus of future work on the evolutionary ecology of survival here and also the focus of attention by public health workers in Botswana.

Other evidence of preference

In 1990 Harpending and Jeffrey Kurland carried out additional field-work among Herero. They carried out interviews about preference and measured heights, weights, and skinfolds of several hundred children. The following material is abstracted from a manuscript by Kurland and Harpending (1992) that describes these approaches to understanding the sex difference in mortality that we found in our reproductive histories and population pyramids.

Herero informants of both sexes and all ages denied that there was any preference for a child of either sex. They agreed that all children were gifts of God, they were precious, and the idea of favouring one sex or the other was abhorrent. The women said that 'of course' women are more interested in daughters and that 'of course' men are more interested in sons, but that these interests developed in late childhood.

---

[1] This neglects the binomial coefficient, but these cancel when the ratio of likelihoods is computed.

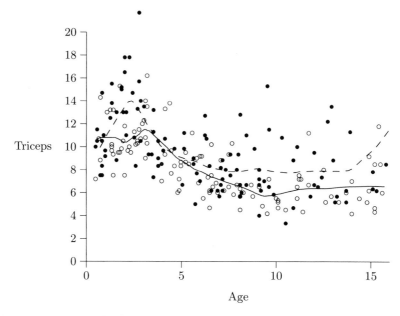

Fig. 3.3. Triceps skinfolds and age among Herero children. The solid line is a lowess regression through the boys' skinfolds, the dashed line is through the girls'. Solid circles are individual female data points, open circles are males

While there was no overt preference, most mothers were aware of the greater frailty of males. They attributed this to two factors. The most important was sorcery: according to them, females are 'nothing' while male infants, who will bring strength to the homestead, the lineage, and the family, are subject to the jealousy and witchcraft of others. This endangers both the child *and the mother*. Several other informants expressed a strong preference for their grandchildren through their daughters, stating that the children of their sons were of 'unknown blood'.

!Kung Bushmen neigbours of the Herero reported that the Herero 'took their daughters to their hearts' and 'refused their sons'. Several !Kung were quite indignant about Herero mistreatment of males and said that the way that Herero treated their little boys was a 'disgrace'. One informant said that she surreptitiously fed a Herero neigbour's male toddler and claimed that without her care he would have died of malnutrition.

When we entered villages we ascertained the whereabouts of all children. Almost without exception the girls not at school were at home, near the women and the food. Boys were away tending animals and cranking wells to water animals. Even boys from 5 to 10 years were away, and both the boys and the men complained at length about the hunger and dangers to which young males but not females were exposed.

In the early morning when 'breakfast' is served at the homestead, girls under 16 were found huddled with their adult female relatives while the boys were off managing cattle at the well. Both Mbukushu indentured workers and Herero boys commonly complained to us about missing the first meal of the day because of labour demands. They also complained about the fact that the girls were always getting 'more food'.

Harpending and Kurland carried out an anthropometric survey of 340 Herero children, reasoning that any sex differential in treatment might leave a signature in growth and development. They found a pattern in the pattern of triceps skinfolds that is unlike any reported in the literature. Females put on a lot of fat after weaning, while the skinfolds of males decline slightly. At age 2 Herero girls have 14 mm of triceps skinfold, males only 10. The difference in the skinfolds between male and female toddlers is highly significant. We do not take these differences to suggest malnutrition of males, but they do confirm the reports of the !Kung and the evidence of mortality rates that Herero take much more diligent care of their daughters. Fig. 3.3 shows the triceps skinfold data points with lowess regression lines through the males and the females. The pattern of fat accumulation in girls in early childhood has not been reported in other populations.

While the pattern of fat growth provides biological confirmation of the sex difference in treatment it does not provide much insight into causes. This evidence pertains to early childhood, while the greatest differential mortality occurs in infancy. Infancy and the treatment of infants, especially in the first few months, is much less visible. Mothers spend the first few months after a birth in rather strict seclusion in a hut with the baby, emerging, covered with blankets or sheets, only for latrine functions or to take the baby to a clinic for immunization.

Conclusions

The patterns derived from percentage of dead offspring by age of mother, tabulations from reproductive histories, and the age–sex structure of the living population are all concordant. Male mortality is much higher than that of females in the last several decades but not before. The difference appeared among children born in the late 1950s and later in terms of off-spring cohorts, and among offspring of women born in the mid-1930s and later, in terms of mothers' cohort.

A model of asymmetric helping between siblings explained properties of the data that were already known but new predictions were only weakly supported by the data. Logistic regression showed that mortality in both sexes was predicted by mortality of older siblings. This suggested heterogeneity among mothers in the survival of all their children. Direct tests for maternal heterogeneity were highly significant for both sons and daughters.

One implication of our findings is that demographers and biologists cannot take cultural norms very seriously as guides to behaviour. Cultural beliefs are statements that informants make to each other (and to anthropologists), that is they are beliefs that are broadcast to others. But if articulated cultural beliefs are more like advertising than they are like simple reflections about motivations that guide behaviour, as some have suggested (e.g. Harpending *et al.* 1987), then understanding behaviour and understanding beliefs are two different problems that are only tenuously related. This point of view runs counter to a trend in demography to incorporate ethnographic methods and information (Caldwell *et al.* 1988).

The Herero expressed no sex preference for their offspring to us, and sex preference is absent generally in Botswana. Yet there are sex differentials as strong as or stronger than in south Asia. Analysis of demographic data shows that in both cases sex preferential treatment has strong effects, in favour of sons in Asia and daughters in Botswana. A task for ethnographic theory is to explain why sex preference is articulated and publicly broadcast in the one context and either unconscious or not articulated in the other.

Until there is a sophisticated theory of overt vs covert beliefs, ethnography does not offer demographers as much as it ought to. Why is the preference for males in south Asia overt, public, and broadcast to others, while the preference for females is covert and perhaps unconscious among the Herero? We have some speculative suggestions.

Speculations

In the Asian case people are typically practising labour intensive plough agriculture, and males are heavily, sometimes exclusively, involved in the work. Marriages are durable and of great economic significance to the participants and their families. While the lives of young women are often unpleasant and difficult, things improve later in the life course as older women acquire political and economic power over their households and younger women within them. There is a sort of reversal of the typical mammalian pattern in which females are the investing sex and males the competitive sex. Here agricultural land and labour limit reproduction as opposed to the female capacity to gestate and lactate. Families compete with other families to buy their daughters into the system of reproduction (Dickemann 1979; Gaulin and Boster 1990).

In these systems husbands and wives have common reproductive interests. Monogamy, the incorporation of women into the families of their husbands, and the relative separation of women from their families of birth mean that husbands and wives share identical benefits and costs of decisions about survival and reproduction of their offspring. Daughters will each require large investments of wealth to enter the reproductive system, and there will be little or no hope of buying more than one or two daughters into marriages. Boys, on the other hand, will provide agricultural labour and their marriages, if they marry, will generate income or at least will be cost free.

Among Herero and among many other sub-Saharan people the ecology of reproduction is quite different (Draper 1989). Durable monogamy is not the most common system of mating, and marriages are not durable. Husbands and wives, lovers, even brothers and sisters do not share common reproductive interests. The interests of Herero men focus on their herds, their *otuzo* (patrilineages), and most important their homesteads and the collection of their dependents in them. Herero women, on the other hand, are focused on 'blood' and on their *omaanda* (matrilineages). The sex difference in the character of responses is striking to us as interviewers—it is as if Herero men had read Durkheim while the women had read Darwin.

This absence of shared interests is probably part of the explanation for the lack of public acknowledgment of preference. If females have a strong preference for daughters or if they are anxious and fear witchcraft when they have sons, then it is not to be shared with men, whose interests and preferences may be quite different.

But this doesn't address the issue of the origins and maintenance of the preferential treatment of daughters by the women. Is there an ecological or economic explanation? Two were suggested to us by Herero women whom we interviewed. One model is that women are considering grandparental investment in their later years, the second is that fear of sons is the result of manipulative ideology maintained by cultural transmission.

The infertility that affected Herero along with many African peoples led to small completed family sizes, a high prevalence of primary sterility, and truncated reproductive careers such that generation time was much shorter in the past. In Chapter 10 we show that generation time has changed from 22 years in the past to 29 years after the population-wide recovery from infertility. Roughly speaking then, a new-born's mother's mother was 44 years old in the past while she is 58 years old today. The life course of women was certainly affected by these demographic facts. Herero theory and practise is that women give birth to children early in the reproductive life course and foster many of these children to other women. Later in the life course women accept foster children from others, especially from their daughters (see Chapter 8). Parental investment and fertility are not so closely coupled in time as they are in many other societies.

Under this regime a woman can plan on expending much of her parental effort on grandchildren. In this context the remarks that women have made to us that the children of their daughters are of their own 'blood' while the children of their sons may be of 'unknown blood' become more salient.

Daughters' children will be opportunities for investment, sons' children will not. An implication of this model is that there should be no preference for grandchildren of either sex, and indeed there is no mortality differential in our data between fostered and non-fostered children.

The second model that may explain the preference for sons is that fear of male infants is a culturally transmitted and maintained manipulative ideology (Krebs and Dawkins 1984; Boyd and Richerson 1985). The prototype of this kind of phenomenon is the pervasive fear of women found among men in the highlands of New Guinea (Harpending *et al.* 1987). Here men tell other men that women are dangerous, polluting, and the source of great danger. It is much safer to avoid women entirely, or at least as long as possible. It is easy to imagine how such a system of beliefs is reproductively advantageous to individual males—if male A can convince male B to avoid women then male A can reproduce at the expense of B. Harpending *et al.* suggested that such an ideology could spread and affect everyone by a 'runaway' process similar to that proposed by R. A. Fisher to explain the spread of individually disadvantageous sexually selected traits like the tails of peacocks. According to this model the fear of witchcraft and sorcery that women with male infants report is, like the fear of women in New Guinea, a culturally transmitted elaboration of reproductive competition that has spread to affect everyone in a maladaptive way.

4
Mortality after early childhood

Introduction

This chapter is a description of mortality rates after childhood among the Herero. The system of year names described in Chapter 1 and our informants' knowledge of family history allowed us to ascertain years of birth and death of many parents, grandparents, and siblings of people whom we interviewed. Using new methods for computing life tables from incomplete lifetimes, we are able to describe adult mortality with a precision that is not ordinarily attainable in anthropological demography. We will give life tables separately for males and females for the years before 1966, which we will call the *early period*, and for 1966 through 1986, the *recent period*.

Herero mortality is relevant to several questions in anthropology and demography. The Herero live in the same environment as the !Kung Bushmen described by Howell (1976; 1979). Compared to !Kung, the prosperous Herero have more food available to them and the food stream is more reliable. There are large herds of cattle and goats buffering them from environmental uncertainty. The difference between the !Kung and Herero life tables suggests that the effect of nutritional status on mortality is strong (see Chapter 9).

The pattern of risk of death by age among the Herero is different from the pattern characteristic of European populations. In comparison to European populations with comparable expectations of life, late middle-aged and old Herero enjoy low risks of death while infants, children, and young adults suffer higher risks. American Black mortality differs from that of American Whites (Manton and Stallard 1984) in the same way. A similar pattern has also been found in census and survey data from central Africa (Gage 1989).

The populations of much of central Africa have been affected by pathological sterility in this century (Frank 1983). Is this an old disorder in this part of the world, or is it recent, having been introduced by outsiders? Has it contributed to or even been the principal cause of the relatively low population densities at contact in central Africa? A common view (Caldwell and Caldwell 1983) is that it must be recent because mortality rates in rural Africa before the Second World War were so high that, in the face of low fertility, African populations would have disappeared. We will suggest that mortality in rural Africa in the past was not as high as others have suggested.

Our life tables are constructed from lifetime information on the off-spring of people that we interviewed and from left-truncated partial life-times of other relatives of our subjects. Combining these two kinds of data is straightforward, but we have not seen it done by anthropologists (but see Hill and Hurtado 1991). Our techniques are applicable to information collected from relatively intense studies of ethnographic or other targeted samples of populations. They take advantage of available details about lifetimes of individuals in a pedigree.

Our methods are not applicable to census and other survey information where there is not much detail obtained from each informant. On the other hand, intensive retrospective studies like ours are done in epidemiology and in historical demography. If, for example, an individual enters a community by marriage, and her death is later recorded, then she provides life table information only from her age at entry or *ascertainment* until her death. This is a *left-truncated* lifetime. Truncation must be accommodated in life table construction.

Issues in adult mortality

Heterogeneity

Many censuses pool information from a diversity of ethnic and class groups, so that published data available for standard demographic analysis repre-sent a heterogeneous mixture of numbers from different underlying pro-cesses. Unique characteristics of subpopulations are blended and buried in this averaging process. While everyone is aware of the potential effects of population heterogeneity, it is nevertheless easy to adopt habits of thought that understand heterogeneity in terms of some underlying average plus the effects of ethnic group or social class or whatever covariate. This statistical framework is very different from an ethnographic framework that seeks to understand the dynamics of demographic processes within relatively homo-geneous subgroups.

The ethnographic point of view suggests that the relatively uniform patterns of survival in human populations are due in part to the blurring of subgroup differences that occurs when data from many groups are pooled, as they are, for example, in national censuses. Life history traits are subject to both biological evolution and cultural evolution, the argument goes, and we ought to try to understand group differences and their evolution.

Biological evolution should affect the trade-off between the 'r-strategy' of an organism that makes many copies of itself at the cost of the quality of the copies and the 'K-strategy' of an organism that makes fewer copies but invests more time, energy, and perhaps risk in each so that they are of higher 'quality', which in evolutionary biology means greater competitive ability. In an algebraic treatment of the trade-off between $r-$ and $K-$strategies, Armstrong and Gilpin (1977) found that the $r-$strategy is favoured by density independent mortality. High mortality rates that are not ameliorable by parental investment should promote the evolution of high fertility, especially early fertility, at the expense of later durability of the organism. Childhood mortality due to infectious agents such as malaria fulfills the conditions of the Armstrong and Gilpin model, while mortality due to malnutrition at weaning is an example of ameliorable mortality, in the sense that higher levels of parental investment can reduce the risk.

Cultural transmission of mating systems and of patterns of parental investment generates differences between human groups but the dynamics of cultural evolution are poorly understood. Pennington and Harpending (1988) and Harpending *et al.* (1990) outline a theory of parental investment and how it might interact with other culturally transmitted behaviours. Their conclusions are similar to those of the ecological model of Armstrong and Gilpin, i.e. that mortality from care-independent causes favours low levels of parental investment in offspring and high fertility. A review of these issues is given in Harpending *et al.* (1987). These models, however, are based on optimization. Many doubt that cultural transmission leads in general to optimum individual behaviour.

The implication of the ethnographic point of view is that statistical analysis of aggregated data is as likely as not to obscure interesting relationships. According to the ethnographic perspective everyone and every group, at least potentially, is facing a different ecology or pursuing some different strategy. Pooled data are an accumulation of facts sampled from a heterogeneous sample space. The difficulty with this point of view is that it is usually unworkable since there can be no meaningful statistical inference from what are essentially anecdotes. And many behaviours, such as cigarette smoking, that influence rates are hardly comprehensible in the strategizing framework.

The statistical framework for thinking about demographic data acknowledges that individuals and families are all different, but it aspires to control these differences by looking at covariates, proxy measures of the underlying causes. For example, income might be taken as a proxy measure of the unobservable social class of a family, or blood pressure, glucose tolerance, and skin wrinkling might be proxies for biological age.

There are also drawbacks to the statistical approach to demography. First, there is usually no real theory about the covariates in the sense of theory being a set of prior hypotheses built from a model of dynamics of a process. Because of this, statistical demography is of great interest and importance to planners, public health and government workers, and businesses but it has not been of so much interest to biologists (Hill and

Hurtado 1991).

Another drawback to the statistical approach is that there is a trade-off between data quantity and data quality. Sampling problems are of little or no concern when census data with information about every individual in a nation of some millions of people are analysed. But these data are hardly ever reliable, and an important concern in demography is how to detect and adjust bad data (Brass *et al.* 1968).

There is a kind of uncertainty principle underlying all of this. We can obtain much low quality information and worry about adjusting away interesting deviations from established norms, or we can obtain a little bit of high quality data and worry about whether patterns in it reflect sampling fluctuations. The tension between these two approaches is the same as the tension between clinicians and epidemiologists in public health, and there are no simple answers to the dilemma. The problem is that demography is not an experimental science, and many of these problems cannot be resolved without experimentation. Kish (1987) provides an interesting discussion of issues of this kind.

We try to walk a middle ground in this chapter. The Herero are relatively homogeneous economically and culturally, in the sense that no one is very poor, everyone lives in about the same kind of hut and eats about the same kind of food, and everyone has access to about the same kind of medical care. Herero have a keen sense of their own ethnicity and they are distinct from other ethnic groups in north-western Botswana both in their own view and in the view of outsiders. By focusing on demographic rates and covariates within Herero we have in principle limited the range of cultural variation in our sample. We also tried to get large numbers of informants so that we could have some assurance that patterns that we found would be statistically meaningful.

Mortality crossover

In North America the mortality rates of Blacks are higher than those of Whites until late adulthood, when a crossover in hazard or annual risk of death occurs. Manton and Stallard (1984, Chapter 5) analyse 1969 mortality data for US White and Black populations and present the age specific hazards of death for each group. Fig. 4.1 shows these rates summed over 5-year intervals. The hazards for Whites of both sexes appear to increase smoothly, like exponential functions, from about age 40. The hazard for Black females increases more slowly in the interval between age 60 and 70, and it crosses the hazard for White females around age 70 or 75. That is to say, a Black woman has a lower risk of death each year after age 75 than does a White woman. The hazard for Black males crosses the hazard for White males in a similar way.

It is troubling that the denominators that Manton and Stallard use to

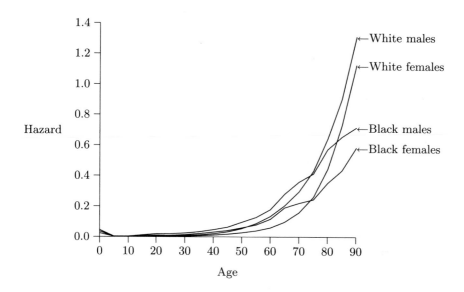

Fig. 4.1. Estimates of the hazard of death by race and sex in the US in 1969. From Tables 2 through 5 in Chapter 5 of Manton and Stallard (1984). The hazard is their 'five year cumulative force of mortality', an estimate of the instantaneous death rate when time is measured in units of 5 years

estimate rates had to be 'adjusted' to account for poor data. While they have faith that the number of deaths of, say, 67-year-old White females in 1969, was reported correctly, a rate estimate is constructed by dividing these deaths by the adjusted population of 67-year-old White females in 1969. The adjustments were made using coefficients given by Siegel (1974). The overall magnitudes of these adjustments were 1.4 per cent for White females, 2.5 per cent for White males, 5.5 per cent for Black females, and 9.9 per cent (!) for Black males.

A popular explanation for the hazard crossover between Blacks and Whites is heterogeneity selection. The argument is that in any population there is some underlying distribution of frailty among individuals and that a given level of environmental insult will be fatal to an individual in proportion to his or her underlying frailty. The environment in childhood and early adulthood was so favourable for Whites and so dangerous for Blacks that, by late middle age, only the hardiest Blacks have survived while many White survivors of moderate and high frailty remain alive because they have not been exposed to dangerous environmental insult. Under comparable environmental conditions, then, middle-aged and old Blacks live longer because they are a hardier subset of the initial distribution. The heterogeneity model does not have strong support from historical data. Old people in, say, England at the turn of the century did not enjoy especially favourable mortality rates although their birth cohort was subject to very high death rates in infancy and childhood.

Another possibility is that there are group differences in life history characteristics that reflect evolution in past environments and that the crossover is a biological property of the population survivor schedule. This hypothesis was suggested by the work of Gage (1989) in which he fit model survival schedules to human mortality data from a world sample of published empirical life tables. Gage found a pattern in national level data from central Africa that was similar to that of American Blacks. Are there fundamental differences in the nature of senescence between races? If there are, why are they present? Do they reflect selective effects of past biological and social environments?

There has been doubt expressed in the demographic literature about the existence of any crossover at all (e.g. Kitigawa and Hauser 1973). For example, if there is undercounting of young adult Black Americans and overcounting of old Black Americans, then the estimates of annual probabilities of death obtained by dividing the number of deaths by the number alive would be systematically biased. Death rates would be over-estimated for young adults and under-estimated for old adults.

Our own mortality analysis is different in kind, being based on truncated lifetimes of people in the past. If we also find a pattern of elevated hazard in early adulthood in comparison to that expected for late adulthood then it will imply that the pattern is real, no matter what its causes may be.

Population dynamics in African history

The quality of data that we have about mortality in Africa in the past is best from those areas where there was a substantial European colonial presence. Colonial governments not only carried out censuses, they also drilled wells and introduced sanitation, health care, police services, and other mortality-reducing programmes. Vaccination and other public health measures improved high death rates that existed before the colonial era. The best information is from West Africa (Brass *et al.* 1968; Hill and Hill 1988) where mortality is extraordinarily high, probably because of marginal nutrition, measles, and high endemicity of malaria. It is not so clear that these conditions are ancient nor that they are characteristic of much of the rest of the continent. Population densities are low throughout much of central Africa's infertility belt (Frank 1983), and consequently nutritional status is probably better. There is, for example, no trace of the mortality peak at 2–3 years of age that is usually attributed to weaning malnutrition in West Africa (Rosetta and O'Quigley 1990).

We will see in Chapter 5 that Herero fertility was very low before the introduction of antibiotics in the late 1950s and that infertility extends as far back in time as our data allow us to see. How old is African infertility? Caldwell and Caldwell (1983) reason that it must be recent, perhaps introduced by Europeans or Arabs, since if it were ancient the affected populations would have died out. This argument assumes that mortality rates in rural Africa were so high that even stationarity required high fertility rates. But if the high mortality assumption is incorrect, then infertility could be an old indigenous disorder in this region and an important factor in understanding the history of central Africa.

Model mortality patterns

Coale-Demeny and Brass models

Standards for human age-specific patterns of mortality are given in model life tables, the best known of which are the Coale and Demeny (1983) series and the relational tables developed by William Brass (Brass 1975; Newell 1988; see also United Nations 1983 and Weiss 1973). These sets of model tables are empirical summaries of the experience of populations from which high quality statistics were available. They were modern populations living under strong central governments with medical care, vaccination, and other public health measures.

There are two ways to view model life tables. First, a model life table can provide a kind of mirror with which to describe an observed survivor schedule. Deviations from a best fitting model are taken to be worthy of comment. Second, the strong uniformitarian position is that a model life table is the 'real' table underlying any set of data, that the data only provide an estimate of the table, and that deviations from the generic human pattern are scarce and demand very strong evidence to be credible. Howell (1979) provides a clear statement of the uniformitarian hypothesis.

Anthropologists should approach the uniformitarian hypothesis with caution. We may use model tables as a set of null hypotheses against which to test data from technologically primitive or ecologically unusual populations. But there is no good theoretical understanding of why mortality risks by age should follow the models since they are only curves fit to data, not models based on a theory of life histories and senescence.

There are several well known deviations from the standard model life tables. One such deviation, for example, is the high ratio of childhood to infant mortality associated with endemic malaria, malnutrition, measles, and alloparental care in parts of West Africa (Brass et al. 1968). The high ratio of male to female infant and childhood mortality that we have found in Herero (see Chapter 3) is not accommodated in the Coale and Demeny series, in which the hazard ratio between the sexes in infancy and childhood is always less than about 1.25 in absolute value. We should remain open to the possibility that other age and sex specific patterns of hazard may exist under ecological circumstances radically different from those of the populations from which model tables were derived.

On the other hand, anthropologists often have small data sets that are of poor quality. In many populations people do not know their own ages nor the years of birth of themselves and their relatives. Ages are assigned by educated guess, although these guesses may be based on careful data management like rank-ordering everyone by age and attempting to anchor the ranking to well known events in the past.

Archaeologists are even worse off. They work with samples of the dead, skeletal populations, rather than the living, and their problems both of ageing and of interpretation are much worse than those presented by living populations. It is perhaps no accident that the strongest claims for qualitatively different life tables have come from the analysis of paleodemographic material (Lovejoy *et al.* 1977; Weiss 1973; Wood *et al.* 1992).

A parametric model

Gage (1989) fit a parametric model to life tables from several published sources. He used the Siler model, which specifies that the hazard of death is composed of three additive components: an exponentially declining hazard that represents infant and childhood mortality, a constant hazard that represents non-senescent hazard like accidental death, and an exponentially increasing hazard that represents senescent changes.

Specifically, the Siler model of the hazard at age x is

$$h(x) = a_i e^{-b_i x} + a_r + a_s e^{b_s x}.$$

There are five parameters in this model, three a's and two b's, so it provides a versatile formalism for describing details of survivor functions.

Gage used a clustering program to group the fitted life tables into five categories or 'types' based on the pattern of change in hazard with age. Overall severity of mortality was removed by regression before the cluster analysis was done. One of the distinct types, his type 3, was represented by populations from sub-Saharan Africa and one Asian population. The distinctive feature of this type was the elevated survival of adults after middle age relative to the other types.

Gage remarked that his type 3 life table was also characteristic of the American Black population, a pattern that has been ascribed to frailty selection. But Gage's finding raises the possibility that this pattern of senescence may be a genetic characteristic rather than an artefact of high early mortality. One might argue that if it were a genetic trait it should have been noticed in other African data, but the quality of information about the ages of old people in Africa is probably so poor that it would be difficult to find a subtle pattern such as this in most published demographic material. The Herero system of year names and our life tables constructed from partial lifetimes provide a unique set of data with which to examine the possibility that comparatively favourable survival schedules in late middle age and old age are characteristic of African populations.

Methods

Life table estimates of survivorship

In this section we describe how we use pedigree information, information about parents and grandparents of informants, to estimate adult mortality. This task must be approached with caution. We could not, for example, simply treat all individuals as a cohort and calculate standard life table statistics since individuals are ascertained at various ages. The nature of the information available about different categories of individuals requires that each be handled differently.

Reproductive histories provide information about the lifetimes of offspring from birth until the time of the interview, when the lifetimes of living children are censored. But other categories of people for whom information is available, like parents of informants, contribute information only from the time that they were ascertained until either their year of death or until we interviewed someone about them. These left-truncated partial lifetimes can be used along with the data from reproductive histories to compute synthetic life tables that pool all available data in an efficient way.

The best way to make clear how we have tabulated data for constructing survivor curves is to provide an extended example. Suppose that we interview a woman, our informant, who was born in 1926. She reports that she had three births, one in 1943, one in 1945, and one in 1948. The first born died in infancy while the other two are alive today. The first birth enters our life table as an infant death in 1943, contributing one person year of life and one death. In effect, we assume that all deaths occur at the end of a year.

Her other two children contribute one person year each at each age until their respective ages in 1986 when our survey was carried out. The second born contributes 41 person years to our life table, and his lifetime is censored since he was still alive when we interviewed his mother. The last born contributes 38 years before censoring.

Since we have aggregated our data into two periods, the lifetimes of individuals may contribute to either one or both periods. Person years before 1966 are our *early* period, while the years 1966 and later are the *recent* period. The second born child of our informant lived from 1945 to 1986, so he contributes 20 person years to the early period life table (i.e. from 1945 to 1965) and 21 to the recent one (from 1966 to 1986). The last born contributes 17 person years to the early period tabulation and 21 to the recent.

Suppose further that our informant reports that the father of her first birth was born in 1906 and that he died in 1970. We say that he was *ascertained* in 1943 at age 37, that is 1943 less 1906. He provides no information about the survival of his cohort from 1906 to 1943, but we assume that he is a random representative of 37-year-olds in 1943 and we enter his person years into our life table from 1943 (age 37) until 1970 (age 64) when he died. He contributes 22 person years to our early life table and is censored at age 59 (i.e. 1965), then he contributes 5 years to the recent life table and contributes a death at age 64 in 1970. The information about his lifetime is said to be *left truncated*.

We used years of the birth of children and years of marriage as events to mark the ascertainment of adults who appeared in reproductive history interviews. There were many individuals ascertained through the birth of children and relatively few ascertained by year of marriage. Herero don't bother to remember the years of marriage and divorce. These events seem quite insignificant in the lives of people, while the births and deaths of relatives are marked very clearly.

Does this indirect ascertainment of partial lifetimes introduce bias? We believe that we might over-estimate maternal mortality of women, that is mortality associated with childbirth, but that otherwise the method is unbiased.

Consider two hypothetical women born in 1920. Woman A had one child in 1940 and then died several years later without having any other children. Woman B had four children, in 1940, 1942, 1944, and 1948, and was still alive in 1986. Assume that all these children survived and are potential informants in our study. If we, in the worst case, were sampling a small fraction of all Herero then we would be four times as likely to include Woman B in our tabulation of indirectly ascertained individuals because she has four children, any one of whom we might interview, while woman A has only one child who is a potential informant.[1]

It seems that our tabulation is biased in favour of high survivorship since we are more likely to ascertain woman B, who lived, than we are to ascertain woman A, who died after only one birth. But woman B contributes person years *only* from the year of birth of the index child to 1986. We are as likely to encounter either child born in 1940, the offspring of woman A or the offspring of woman B. If instead we encounter another of B's children, say the third born, woman B enters our tabulation at age 24 (i.e. 1944 less 1920), and her person years from 1940 to 1944 are not entered. So we

---

[1] If we encountered and interviewed woman B herself then she provides no information about her own survival and her lifetime is not entered into the life table unless she was independently ascertained through one of her children.

are indeed more likely to ascertain high fertility parents, but if we assume that survival and fertility are uncorrelated then we do not over-estimate survival. Our method is not biased in favour of low mortality.

We are not happy with the assumption of uncorrelated fertility and mortality but we have no strong evidence that fertility either increases or decreases future mortality. The current cohort of old people suffered from very low fertility in their reproductive years. Many of them have no surviving children today, yet old people are treasured and well taken care of by Herero. Families and familial obligations are strong, and all old people are taken in by relatives, although these relatives are sometimes genealogically quite distant.

On the other hand, we were often told by Herero that the most important determinant of a good old age is the existence of offspring of both sexes who can provide care. The Herero model suggests that individuals who had no or few offspring would receive worse care in their late adulthood and old age and might indeed suffer higher hazards of death. If their model is correct then our adult mortality estimates are biased in favour of low hazard rates. However, we never observed any relationship between the quality of care that old people received and the numbers of their children. More important determinants of quality of care seemed to be the numbers of children available in the homestead to run errands and provide services.

We do know that fertility increases mortality in women during the reproductive years. There were a few deaths in childbirth and immediately after childbirth reported to us. Our estimates of female mortality in the 20–30-year-old women may be biased upward by this maternal mortality. Many women never had a live birth because of the prevalence of pathological sterility in the past. These women were not subject to the danger of childbirth, of course, and neither could they be named by children who would become our informants. Only fertile women could be ascertained by us a generation later.

A more worrisome source of bias is missing data: there were some informants who did not know the birth years of one or, occasionally, both parents. Tabulations revealed that people whose birth years were unknown were more likely to be dead, raising the possibility that our data were systematically biased in favour of living parents, leading to under-estimation of mortality rates in adulthood. But another tabulation revealed that the number of times a person was mentioned by informants was the best predictor of whether his or her year of birth was known. The years of birth of old people, alive or dead, who were named in four or five different interviews were usually known by at least one or two of our informants. The birth years of people mentioned in a single interview, on the other hand, were least likely to be known.

As a check on this potential source of bias we entered parents with

Table 4.1. Numbers of person years and deaths available for constructing life tables. The cases where year of birth was unknown were allocated according to the empirical distribution of age of parenthood. Early period is before 1966, recent period is 1966–86

		Males		Females	
Early period	Birthyear	yes	no	yes	no
	Person years	12761	1558	13803	1854
	Deaths	242	44	163	28
Recent period	Birthyear	yes	no	yes	no
	Person years	17459	1267	19355	1255
	Deaths	240	24	164	24

unknown birth years into our life table with the year of birth specified as a probability distribution rather than as a single number. We used the empirical distribution of age at parenthood separately for men and women. For example, assume that an informant was born in 1930 and that she reported that she did not know the year of birth of her mother but that her mother died in 1957. Her mother contributes 27 person years of life and one death to our life table, but since we don't know when she was born we do not know when those years were. Instead we know that 5.8 per cent of mothers of the rest of our informants were age 20 when the informant was born, 6.6 per cent were age 21, etc. Following this distribution, we enter 5.8 per cent of a single individual into our life table as having been born in 1910 and ascertained at age 20, 6.6 per cent of a person as having been born in 1909 and ascertained at age 21, etc. In this way, we avoid the possibility that we are biasing our adult mortality estimates toward high adult survivorship by preferentially including parents who are alive. Table 4.1 shows the total numbers of person years and of recorded deaths that we have for each of our four life tables, separated into those for whom we knew the year of birth and those for whom it was unknown. We refer to lifetimes that were allocated over a distribution of possible birth years as *imputed* lifetimes.

We discuss these augmented life tables in the rest of this chapter, but we point out that the addition of the imputed person years made no visible difference in the patterns that we found. Survivor functions from augmented and non-augmented life tables were nearly indistinguishable.

Constructing the survivor function

The survivor function of a life table at age x is the probability that a person will survive from the age of entry to age x. It is conventionally written l_x

to mean the probability of surviving from birth to age x or greater. We will also present some estimates of conditional survivor functions. For example, the maternal orphanhood method described below estimates the probability that a woman survived from age 25 to age x, written $_{25}l_x$.

The survivor functions that we describe in this chapter were constructed by pooling the left truncated lifetimes described above, the full lifetimes of offspring of informants, and the imputed lifetimes of parents whose exact years of birth were not known. All these categories of lifetime may be right censored, that is the individual may have been alive in 1986.

The age of ascertainment of an individual is the age at which the (oldest) informant that is an offspring of that parent was born, in the case of children telling us about their parents. Individuals ascertained through co-parenthood or marriage with an informant enter our tabulation at the earliest year at which they were ascertained. That year is treated as a whole year of life. We assume that births occur at the end of the year. We also assume that both deaths and censoring occur at the end of a year, so that the estimated hazard q_x of death at each age x is the number of deaths at age x divided by the sum of the number of parents who lived through age x, the number who were censored at age x, and the number of deaths at age x.

The survivor function l_x is then computed as the *product limit* estimate (Kaplan and Meier 1958)

$$l_x = \prod_{i=0}^{x-1}(1 - q_i).$$

Confidence limits for the estimated survivor function l can be computed by the formula given in Kalbfleisch and Prentice (1980, p. 15 ff.), and two estimated curves can be compared using the log-rank test described on pages 16 ff. of the same reference.

We have computed estimated survivorship functions for males and females separately, to examine sex differences in mortality, and for person years before and after 1965, to examine temporal trends in mortality. The resulting curves refer neither to any single discrete time nor to any single cohort of parents. The oldest parent was born in 1846, while offspring of informants could have been born as recently as 1986 and still contribute a person year to the data.

Our interest is to generate estimates rather than to test hypotheses, so statistical tests about our findings are not of great relevance save that they provide an indication of the reliability of the differences we find. For example, the log-rank test for the overall difference between the male survivor functions in the early and recent periods against the hypothesis that they reflect the same mortality experience is $X_1^2 = 12.9$, a highly significant dif-

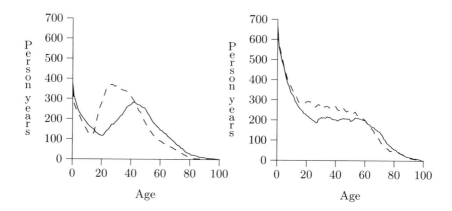

Fig. 4.2. Number of person years available for estimating survivor functions and hazards. The left panel shows person years in the early period (before 1966), the right panel shows person years in the recent period (1966–86). Males are the solid lines, females the dashed lines

ference. The corresponding statistic for the difference between males and females in the early period is 6.8, with an associated probability of less than 0.01.

Fig. 4.2 shows the number of person years available at each age and for each sex and period. These numbers are the denominators, at each age, for the estimated hazard of death. The strange shapes of these curves reflect the two different sources of data; informants' reports about their own children provide person years from birth onward, while information about parents of informants is concentrated in the 20s and 30s for mothers and the 30s and 40s for fathers. The dip in person years of teenagers in the early period is a consequence of the infertility of that period. There were simply not many births, and we do not start to pick up person years about parents until the ages of twenty and greater for mothers and thirty and greater for fathers.

These tabulations show that we have the most information about adults in the early period and about childhood in the recent period. In all cases the data are quite sparse past age 70 and inference about rates at this age and greater is not very reliable.

The estimates of the survivor function for 5-year intervals are in Table 4.2. They are plotted by single year in Fig. 4.3. Males and females are shown separately for the early and recent periods in both the table and the figure.

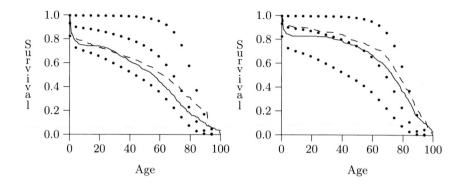

Fig. 4.3. Unsmoothed survivor functions. The early period (before 1966) is the left panel and the recent period (1966–86) is the right panel. The solid line is males, the dashed line females. The three series of bullets are survivor curves from the Coale and Demeny (1983) model West series of life tables, the bottom series corresponding to $\overset{\circ}{e}_0=40$ years, the middle to $\overset{\circ}{e}_0=60$ years, the top to $\overset{\circ}{e}_0=80$ years.

Smoothing by logistic regression

It is more informative to look directly at estimates of the hazard at each age implied by a life table than it is to look at the survivor function. The attraction of the survivor function is that it is smooth, while the hazard is jagged and irregular in small samples. On the other hand, the hazards at each age are independent while the survivor function reflects all the mortality at earlier ages. Survivor curves are difficult to compare by eye. It is possible to smooth the hazard function yet retain its important features.

In many applications of hazard analysis a parametric function is fit to the observed hazards, for example functions that specify a constant hazard, a hazard that changes linearly or exponentially, a bathtub-shaped hazard that might be appropriate for the whole human life-span, etc. Our interests are not so much in fitting an a priori model as they are in simply smoothing the jagged hazard to obtain a better visual idea of its shape. For this modest purpose logistic regression is a versatile tool. We have used a procedure described by Efron (1988) in which the logit of the hazard is fit by maximum likelihood to a polynomial function of age.

We write q_x for the hazard at age x, i.e. the probability that an individual at his or her xth birthday will die in the next year, and write λ for the logit of the hazard, i. e.

$$\lambda_x = \ln\left(\frac{q_x}{1-q_x}\right).$$

Table 4.2. Empirical survivor functions (l_x) by sex and period

Age	Early males	Early females	Recent males	Recent females
0	1.000	1.000	1.000	1.000
5	0.773	0.794	0.838	0.912
10	0.745	0.781	0.826	0.901
15	0.741	0.745	0.826	0.898
20	0.740	0.726	0.826	0.892
25	0.724	0.708	0.822	0.867
30	0.694	0.684	0.821	0.860
35	0.649	0.666	0.800	0.849
40	0.611	0.644	0.785	0.841
45	0.583	0.619	0.762	0.802
50	0.542	0.589	0.739	0.782
55	0.503	0.562	0.703	0.766
60	0.439	0.513	0.670	0.729
65	0.375	0.479	0.614	0.709
70	0.309	0.414	0.555	0.644
75	0.237	0.362	0.462	0.541
80	0.175	0.309	0.360	0.442
85	0.145	0.240	0.261	0.325

The logit transformation is convenient because it maps a probability, constrained to be between zero and one, into a number that is unconstrained. A minor problem is that the data points are observed fractions, they can be either zero or one, and the logit of either zero or one is undefined. It is difficult to do logistic regression with conventional least squares routines. Instead, the model is fit by maximum likelihood. For any set of parameter values, we compute the likelihood of the data given these parameters. This likelihood surface has a maximum (optimistically only one) and the parameter values corresponding to the maximum of the likelihood surface are the maximum likelihood estimates. These estimates are found by a numerical procedure that locates the maximum of this surface.

Specifically, the model is

$$\hat{\lambda}_x = \sum_{i=0}^{n} \alpha_i x^i$$

where n is the order of the polynomial. If n is 0 the model corresponds to a constant hazard while if n is 1 this is very close to a Gompertz hazard. Higher order polynomials apparently do not correspond to familiar hazard functions. An attractive feature of this method, besides its simplicity, is that other covariates can be added to the regression without difficulty.

Table 4.3. Changes in the log-likelihood ratio X^2 statistic from adding successive powers of age to the logistic regression. Early period is before 1966, recent period is 1966–86

Term	Early males	Early females	Recent males	Recent females
x	122.2	33.0	233.4	192.6
x^2	1.2	5.4	3.6	18.6
x^3	1.2	0.0	2.0	0.0
x^4	1.0	0.0	2.4	0.0

Since infant and childhood mortality adds complexity to the hazard estimates we have fit the logistic model to our survival data between ages 5 and 100 only. When we include infant and childhood mortality we are forced to fit a fifth degree polynomial and the simplicity that we seek is lost. By restricting our fit to the ages of 5 and greater we have to retain only terms in x^2 to describe the data adequately. Table 4.3 shows how twice the logarithm of the likelihood changes as successively higher powers of age enter the regression. Under the null hypothesis of no improvement, each log-likelihood would be distributed approximately as a χ^2 variable with one degree of freedom. The female hazard curves clearly require that the quadratic term be added while the male hazards are adequately fit by retaining only the linear term, that is they are fit by a Gompertz function. The female rates are clearly not fit by a Gompertz.

Orphanhood methods

Another more standard method for inferring the mortality of adults is to tabulate the percentage of informants of each age who are maternal and paternal orphans. Maternal orphanhood estimates the mortality of females, paternal orphanhood of males. The idea, roughly, is that if half the fathers of 40-year-old informants are dead and if the average age of fathers of these informants was 35 when they were born, then survival from 35 to 75 is about 0.5. In practice various adjustments are made. Tables are provided in United Nations *Manual X* (United Nations 1983) for converting both maternal and paternal orphanhood tabulations to estimates of survivor functions given the average ages of maternity and paternity in the population. In our case orphanhood statistics provide estimates of the survival of mother from age 25 to 40 and greater and of fathers from age 37.5 to age 55 and greater.

Fig. 4.4 shows orphanhood estimates of survivorship for males and females along with segments of the empirical life tables for the early and recent periods. The orphanhood methods do seem to provide reasonable estimates of the mortality of parents of informants in the sense that the

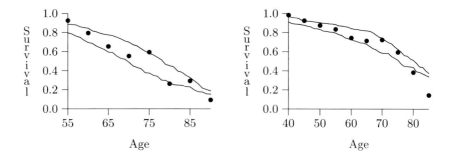

Fig. 4.4. Estimated survival of males from age 37.5 by paternal orphanhood, in the left panel, and of females from age 25, in the right panel. The solid lines are life table estimates for the early (before 1966) and recent (1966–86) periods, while the bullets show the orphanhood estimates.

data points are usually between the more precise estimates for the early and recent periods.

The orphanhood answers are not entirely satisfactory for several reasons. First, there is much variation from one estimate to the next—they do not generate a smooth curve. Second, the orphanhood methods answer questions that we would not otherwise have thought of asking, such as 'what is male survivorship from age 37.5 to age 65?' We think that the implication is that in populations where ages or birth dates are known it is highly preferable for anthropologists to take the time to ask years of birth and death of as many relatives as possible, since such information leads to much better estimates of survivor functions.

Results

Overall mortality

In Fig. 4.3 the estimates of the Herero survivor functions are compared to three Coale and Demeny model West life tables: the lowest series of bullets is of a model population with expectation of life at birth of 40 years, the middle of a model with $\overset{\circ}{e}_0 = 60$ years, and the top series of a model with $\overset{\circ}{e}_0 = 80$ years.

The expectation of life at birth is estimated by summing the survivor function over the whole life-span. These estimates are given in Table 4.4.

The survivor functions show familiar features. Female survivorship is higher than that of males in each period and at all ages except that female mortality in the early period during the early ages of child-bearing was substantial. The survivor function for females briefly crosses that for males in this period in the late teens and early 20s. But recall that the method,

Table 4.4. Expectation of life at birth by period and sex

Early males	Early females	Recent males	Recent females
47.9	52.5	61.9	67.8

relying as it does on reports of children about their parents, over-estimates mortality associated with child-bearing. Sterile women were not exposed to the hazard of child-bearing, and in older cohorts approximately 15 per cent of women were childless.

A comparison of the left and right panels of Fig. 4.3 shows that adult mortality has improved since the mid-1960s. The survival of females is better than that of males in each period and at all ages save for early adulthood in the early period, when mortality probably associated with childbirth causes the survivor curves to cross. As we mentioned above, this female mortality is exaggerated by our methods and the crossing of the curves is probably not a real phenomenon.

The difference in expectation of life at birth between the early period is approximately 15 years—$\overset{\circ}{e}_0$ for males was 48 in the early period and is 62 in the recent period, while female $\overset{\circ}{e}_0$ has gone from 53 to 68.

Dramatic improvement in infant and childhood mortality is evident in comparing the two panels, as is the failure of male infants and children in the recent period to enjoy the same favourable rates as their sisters. Recent male infant and childhood mortality remains high, while that of females is quite good.

There is a big change in death rates, and we are at a loss to explain it. Today rural areas are served by clinics that provide obstetric and paediatric care, immunizations, and treatment of acute and chronic illnesses. The clinics are well stocked and maintained. Anecdotal reports to us by medical officers in Botswana suggest that the quality of health services in Botswana exceeds that of most if not all sub-Saharan African countries outside South Africa. But these clinics are quite recent, having appeared in the remote north-west, where much of our survey was done, only in the late 1970s. However, widespread vaccination against childhood diseases was introduced much earlier.

There is a trend in both periods for the survivor functions to 'catch up' with the Coale and Demeny model populations at older ages. For example, at age 10 in the early period male survival is like that of a model population with $\overset{\circ}{e}_0=40$, while by age 90 it is surpassing a model with $\overset{\circ}{e}_0=80$. Adult survival is better than it 'ought' to be given the death rates of infants and children. This phenomenon is even more apparent when we look at direct estimates of hazard.

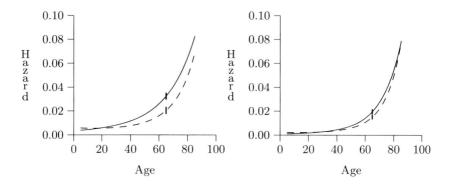

Fig. 4.5. Smoothed estimates of the yearly hazard of death from age 5 to age 80 in the early (left panel) and recent (right panel) periods. The solid line is the hazard to males, the dashed line the hazard to females. Confidence bars two standard errors wide are drawn at age 65. The early period is before 1966, the recent period is 1966–86.

Fig. 4.5 shows the fitted age-specific hazard functions. To avoid clutter we have not drawn the two standard error regions but have only drawn error bars at age 65 for each curve. Each error bar is two standard errors wide. These show that in the early period male adult mortality was very different from that of females while recently the mortality rates of the two sexes seem to have converged. In both periods the two standard error confidence bars are non-overlapping at age 65 but the difference is much greater in the early period. In the early period, confidence intervals are disjoint between ages 30 and 75, in the recent period between 55 and 70 only. The difference in the recent period is probably not reliably different from zero. In both periods the hazards converge in extreme old age, but the data are sparse at these old ages.

Table 4.5 shows the observed and expected numbers of deaths for each life table aggregated into 10-year intervals from 5–15 to 95–105. An indication of goodness of fit of the logistic smoothing is provided by the *deviance* X^2 statistics given in the last row. These should be approximately χ^2 variables with seven degrees of freedom. They show an entirely satisfactory fit.

Late middle and old age

In Fig. 4.6 we show 5-year sums of the annual age specific hazard of death for the 1969 White population of the United States (Manton and Stallard 1984, p. 152) along with the same quantities computed from the Herero

Table 4.5. Observed and expected deaths for each life table, aggregated into 10-year intervals. The X^2 statistics in the bottom row should be distributed approximately as χ_7^2. Early period is before 1966, recent period is 1966–86

	Early males		Early females		Recent males		Recent females	
	obs	exp	obs	exp	obs	exp	obs	exp
5–14	8.0	9.0	8.6	9.1	4.3	6.0	8.0	6.0
15–24	7.5	3.0	14.7	14.3	4.1	1.0	6.6	10.0
25–34	15.2	20.5	22.2	21.9	5.7	5.7	7.4	5.6
35–44	30.5	28.4	23.6	22.6	9.2	10.0	9.7	14.3
45–54	40.2	34.9	19.1	18.5	15.8	16.4	14.4	11.4
55–64	38.3	43.0	14.7	15.4	26.9	25.6	20.7	15.5
55–74	33.3	37.3	13.0	13.9	36.3	37.3	22.2	26.4
75–84	18.7	15.9	5.4	5.3	30.9	32.0	22.1	22.5
85–94	8.7	8.4	1.5	1.8	20.3	19.5	19.8	16.8
95–	2.2	2.3	0.2	0.2	5.3	5.2	4.0	6.3
Totals	202.6	202.6	122.9	122.9	158.7	158.7	134.9	134.9
X^2		7.8		0.3		4.1		9.5

hazards in the recent period.[2]

Herero mortality rates are higher than those of US Whites before age 40–5, but after this age the death rate of White males apparently exceeds that of both Herero males and females. The death rates of US White males and females diverge sharply after the 40s, while the two sexes suffer similar death rates among the Herero.

Taken at face value, these hazard rates imply that Herero male mortality is lower than that of US White males in 1969 past age 45 and that Herero female mortality is lower than that of US females in 1969 past age 60. The US data are based on such large numbers that there is effectively no estimation error, while the standard errors of the estimates of Herero mortality are appreciable. The two standard error confidence limits on the Herero curves are discrete at age 65, but barely so, as was shown in Fig. 4.5. Manton and Stallard (1984) show that in the US data the Black female hazard flattens and diverges from the shape of that of the White population from age 65 or so on while the Black male hazard flattens and

---

[2]Suppose that at the beginning of a year there are N_x individuals age x and that D_x of them die during the year. Then an estimate of the mortality probability for those entering the cohort is $q_x = D_x/N_x$. Manton and Stallard work instead with an estimate of the accumulated hazard over the year under a continuous time model, computed as $h_x = -\ln(1 - q_x)$. The two quantities are almost identical. The hazard is also occasionally estimated by dividing the number of deaths by an estimate of the mid-year population, $N(x)$ less half the deaths that occurred during the year. It is important that these estimators be used consistently but it is of little significance in our context which one is used.

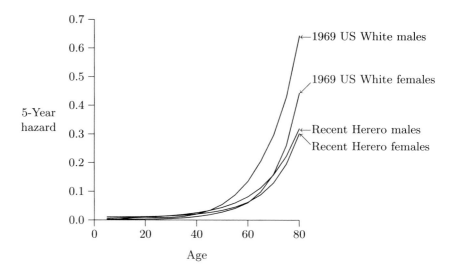

Fig. 4.6. Five-year hazard rates of the male and female US White population in 1969 and of recent (1966–86) male and female Herero. US rates from Manton and Stallard (1984).

diverges past age 85 (see Fig. 2, p. 155, of their monograph). The Herero pattern is qualitatively similar to that of the US Black population but the crossover occurs earlier.

While the details are subject to sampling noise, Herero hazards of death are clearly reliably lower than those of US White males in old age, and they are probably lower than those of US White females in later old age. Is this crossover an effect of high mortality between birth to middle age and heterogeneity selection? If so, such an effect should appear in life tables from other high mortality populations.

The heterogeneity argument is that severe conditions early in the life-span remove the frail end of the distribution of individual frailty, so that those who reach old age are a hardy subset of their birth cohort. The prediction is that high infant and childhood mortality in a cohort will lead to mild mortality rates in old age. An easy check on this prediction is provided by mortality data from the eighteenth and nineteenth century in Europe where high quality census information is available.

Keyfitz and Flieger (1968, pp. 604 ff.) provide life tables for Swedish 5-year cohorts who were 0–4 years of age in 1780 through 1925. We compared male infant mortality and the probability, at age 75, of dying before 80 for the 21 cohorts born from 1780 to 1880. If high infant mortality selects for hardiness in old age, the correlation between these two measures of mortality should be negative. A naïve wear-and-tear model predicts a positive correlation. The actual correlation is +0.81. On the other hand, this positive correlation may mostly reflect the secular trend in mortality in the eighteenth and nineteenth centuries in Europe. The correlation between residuals from exponential trends fitted to the two series is −0.24, providing some support for the heterogeneity selection model of the frailty of the old. Others, such as Caselli and Capocaccia (1989), have also reached ambivalent conclusions about heterogeneity selection.

Conclusions

Our analysis of these historical data on Herero adult mortality do not yield any dramatic surprises apart from the extraordinarily favourable mortality of old people. The effects of age and sex are entirely in accord with expectations from model life tables, the figures in our data corresponding to populations with expectations of life at birth around 50 for our early period (before 1966) sample and around 65 for our recent period (1966–86).

An interesting implication of our results for anthropology is the perspective they give to the population biology of the !Kung Bushmen. Nancy Howell (Howell 1979) has studied the demography of the !Kung who live in the same region of the Kalahari as the Herero that we are studying. Her conclusion was that the !Kung experienced a life table corresponding to an expectation of life at birth of 30 years, which is significantly lower than that of the Herero at around 50 in the past and around 60 recently.[3] These two groups share the same environment and most of the same infectious agents (the Herero, living with cattle, are expected to be more exposed to pathogens), yet Herero survivorship is much better. The Herero are pastoralists who have access to plentiful quantities of milk and meat, while the !Kung are hunter-gatherers who eat a lot of low quality vegetable food. We take the difference in expectation of life to suggest that diet has large effects on survival rates. This evidence contradicts the idea that the !Kung are 'affluent' or that their diet was ever suitable or adequate.

Our findings also challenge the widespread assumption that mortality in rural African populations in pre-contact times was very much higher than it is today. For example, Caldwell and Caldwell (1983) argue that African sterility must be recent because the populations affected would have disappeared in the face of high mortality in the past. But the Herero material suggests that mortality in earlier times need not have been so high, and that population stationarity could have been achieved with total fertility

---

[3] At the end of Chapter 4, Howell discusses the survivorship of people between 1964 and 1973. She finds that the mortality that they experienced was considerably lower than mortality in the past. The chapter concludes with a fitted life table with an expectation of life of 50. It is easy to fail to notice that this final table in her chapter reflects recent experience, not her main findings.

rates of between three and four, i.e. those characteristic of areas severely affected with infertility. The age pattern of mortality among Herero, as in other African populations, is quite different from that of European populations. Infant, childhood, and early adult death rates are high, but the survivors enjoy mild risks of death to ages as old as we can measure.

Speculations

The unexpected shape of the hazard function in old age is, we think, real and not a statistical artefact. It is the sort of finding that would arouse suspicion were it not for the corroborating evidence of the same pattern in the American Black population and other sub-saharan African material discussed by Gage (1989). The extraordinary hardiness of old people in these populations directly contradicts a controversial model of human group differences that has been recently advocated by Rushton (1987).

In a coarse-grained application of the model of the trade-offs between r- and K-strategies to human races, Rushton suggested that of the major races Orientals are relatively the most K-selected while Africans are the most r-selected. Briefly, an r-selected organism devotes resources to reproduction at the cost of the quality of offspring, quality meaning durability and competitive ability. A K-selected organism, on the other hand, sacrifices fertility to making fewer high quality offspring able to compete with conspecifics. Among plants, weeds are r-selected while tropical trees are K-selected. This model is better regarded as an empirical generalization than as a model since there is no proper theory that explains it.

While the idea of a continuum between concentrating on maintenance vs reproduction is appealing, it has been very difficult to develop models that describe this continuum. The Armstrong and Gilpin model that we discussed previously is one of the best, but it does not seem to have led to further work. The r- and K-strategy continuum remains a good idea, but not much more than that. At any rate, it is worth considering Rushton's arguments because there are differences among members of our species that are worth understanding.

Rushton suggests that Orientals are the most K-selected of human races, that Europeans are intermediate, and that Africans are the most r-selected. But the hardiness of the elderly in Black populations is in direct contradiction to Rushton's use of the r–K continuum to fit differences between races. Whatever the differences among human continental groups are, they do not follow the same regularities as the differences among weeds, willows, and teak trees, the prototypical sequence of organisms used to illustrate the continuum. Is the durability of late middle age and old age among African populations a quirk? Are Oriental old even more durable?

Fig. 4.7 shows several populations plotted according to the expectation of life at birth, on the x-axis, and the probability that a 75-year-old male

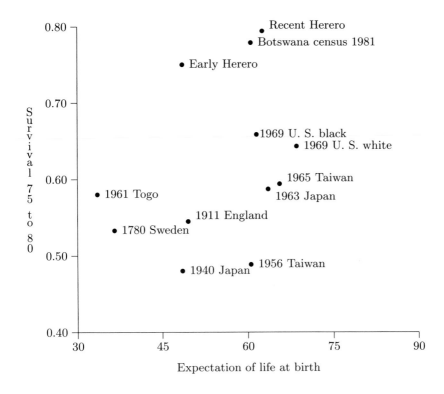

Fig. 4.7. Expectation of life at birth (*x*-axis) and male survival from 75 to 80 (*y*-axis) from various populations. See text for details.

will survive the next 5 years on the *y*-axis. The US Black and White data are from Manton and Stallard (1984), the Herero from the present study, and the others from the census of Botswana and the tabulations of Keyfitz and Flieger (1968). Apparently there is no strong relationship between these two measures of hardiness: the old in high mortality populations may enjoy relatively favourable survival prospects, as in Togo in 1961, or very poor prospects, as in Japan in 1940. The only apparent pattern is that Oriental populations lie in the south-east corner of the plot: for a given expectation of life at birth the hazard of death to old people is very high. Conversely, African populations are in the north-west: for a given expectation of life at birth the hazard of death to old people is low. The relative ranking of the major groups suggested by Rushton seems to hold, but the ranking is *directly opposite* to that suggested by him.

The evolutionary theory of senescence, due to Hamilton (1966),

Williams (1957; 1966), Medawar (1957),, and others is summarized in Charlesworth (1980) and Roughgarden (1979). An organism that does not senesce still dies from other causes, so that genetic modifiers that favour early viability and reproduction can be selected even if they decrease later viability.

An even simpler idea, favoured by Charlesworth, is that selection against deleterious mutations is strongest early in reproductive life and weakest later. Consider, for example, an organism that does not senesce but that experiences a 10 per cent probability of death each year from predation. Very few of them survive until, say, age 15, and there is very weak selection against deleterious mutations that are expressed at age 15. On the other hand there is strong selection against deleterious mutations that have an effect at the beginning of reproduction. These interactions between age, exogenous hazard, and selection lead to the evolution of senescence.

This theory seems too general to provide any help for understanding differences among human groups. It is especially unhelpful in the case of human females, who undergo menopause. The differences among groups that we are considering are differences in hardiness long past the age of menopause.

Two indirect selection pressures (Hamilton 1964; Rogers 1990) might bear on the issue of hardiness of the old. On the one hand, if old people can invest in grandchildren and other kin by providing parental care and perhaps other resources that they control, then selection will favour hardiness of the elderly. On the other hand, if old people compete with children, grandchildren, and other kin for food and other resources then selection will not favour hardiness. Since they are past the age at which they are capable (female) or likely (male) to reproduce, indirect selection will instead favour rapid senescence and failure.

A prediction is that senescence would be favoured in environments where food is chronically scarce and where people live and share food with close kin. If old people are taking food from the mouths of their own children and grandchildren then selection would favour suicidal senescence unless they are able to contribute to the fitness of other members of their family.

The opposite conditions favour hardiness of the elderly. If food is not scarce and if the old people can contribute to the fitness of their kin, perhaps through child-care or through political connections and manipulative ability, then hardiness would be favoured. Hardiness would also be favoured by social systems with households that are not concentrations of closely related individuals. There would be no selective pressure on the old to sacrifice themselves to benefit unrelated individuals.

Does the hardiness of the elderly tell us anything about the ecological circumstances of life history evolution in Africa? Fostering and care of children by grandparents and other old people is very widespread in Africa (see Chapter 8). Old people, especially old women, spend a lot of time 'mothering' fostered in children, especially grandchildren. It is intriguing to speculate that such an allocation of parental effort over the life course, an allocation that seems different from any European norm, might be related to the hardiness of the old. But cause and effect are not so clear; it might be that care of grandchildren has been a selective agent favouring hardiness of the old, or it might be as well that the hardiness of the old favours the allocation of parenting duties to them in a way that would not work in a population subject to a European pattern of senescence.

5

Measures of fertility, past and present

Introduction

Anthropologists and biologists have traditionally been interested in the fertility of populations because the rate of reproduction is one of the two variables that determines how fast they grow, and this in turn reflects success at competiion in their environment. The goal of finding a relationship between subsistence regime and the fertility and mortality of groups has been at the core of much population research in anthropology. Interactions among subsistence system, mortality, and fertility may determine the evolutionary trajectories of groups. During our early history as hunter-gatherers, populations grew slowly, with rates of fertility only marginally offsetting mortality. When humans began adopting agriculture, population growth apparently increased. Disagreement over whether the population expansion was caused by increased fertility or decreased mortality associated with food production and the concomitant sedentary life-style is the subject of a lively debate (Cohen 1989). Because it is believed that we lived in small bands through much of our history, studies of small populations have been particularly relevant to understanding this issue.

More recently human ecologists have turned to theories of individual strategizing and the social and biological costs associated with the reproductive behaviour of individuals. The fertility of individuals and the mortality of themselves and their offspring are tied to factors such as differential access to resources that are in turn related to the health, social status, wealth, marriage choices, and education of individuals in contemporary populations.

We were initially interested in understanding how Herero women modified their reproductive rate in response to their own individual life course events and circumstances. Our analysis of their fertility, however, shows that the Herero have a history of unusually low fertility that predates the turn of this century at least. We believe the reproductive choices of Herero women were so constrained that individual life histories have played an insignificant role.

Herero depopulation was noted earlier in this century, leading to speculation that the Herero were committing 'tribal suicide' by refusing to give birth (Steenkamp 1944; Gibson 1959; Almagor 1982a). Our research suggests, however, that Herero are part of the extensive 'African infertility belt' (Coale 1968; Frank 1983; Caldwell and Caldwell 1983). Like many of the people of central Africa, the Herero, the !Kung, and other groups occupying north-western Botswana, have suffered from a pathological condition that, until recently, significantly reduced their fertility. We suggest that infertility has a long history in Africa and that models of population ecology based on African demographic data may be flawed.

In this chapter we describe a dramatic transition from very low to very high fertility among Herero women. We use several different methods to describe Herero fertility to show that abnormally low reproductive rates predate the turn of the century. First, we present the age-specific fertility rates of women reproducing in four different periods. These rates show that Herero fertility was unusually low throughout the first half of the century but began increasing in the late 1950s. Next, we examine the family sizes of cohorts of post-reproductive women. The cohort rates confirm the trends suggested by the period fertility rates. We then use an indirect method to impute the fertility of the mothers of our informants to extend our examination of trends in Herero fertility further into the past. Finally, we compare the directly and indirectly obtained family size distributions and compute their parity progression ratios to illustrate the onset of sterility in Herero. Altogether our data show that Herero fertility has been low for a long time and that it is currently at its highest level in at least a century.

In the next chapter, we examine potential causes of low Herero fertility and the sudden fertility surge in the 1950s. We focus on the effects of diseases, on the effects of differences in parenting behaviour, and on the effects of health on fertility. We also consider ecological or adaptational constraints on Herero fertility. We show that sterility caused by the sequelae of sexually-transmitted diseases (STDs) is the best explanation for the low Herero fertility. In the last three decades, Herero fertility increased by more than four births per woman as an apparent effect of STD control in north-western Botswana. We also discuss the implications of infertility in Africa for models of human population ecology and African history. We explore these issues further in Chapter 9, where we re-examine the !Kung Bushmen hunter-gatherer demographic model in the context of African infertility and Herero mortality.

Age-specific fertility rates

Definitions

Age-specific fertility rates (ASFRs) show the age pattern of fertility. We computed them by summing the number of births that women had at each age and dividing this sum by how many women were at risk at that age. Demographers compute both period and cohort rates. Period ASFRs measure the fertility of women reproducing during a defined time regardless of when they were born, while cohort ASFRs measure the fertility of women born during a defined time. The total fertility rate (TFR), which is simply the sum of a set of ASFRs, is a convenient summary of fertility for making comparisons between populations or groups of women. The ASFRs estimate the expected number of births to women at each age, and the TFR measures the expected number of births to women during their reproductive span. If fertility is constant through time, the period TFR and the cohort TFR will be equal (Newell 1988).

Demographers often prefer to compute ASFRs from recent rather than retrospectively reported births. Factors such as poor memory recall, underreporting of deceased offspring, and selective maternal mortality may bias rates based on retrospective fertility histories. Few studies report cohort rates since they require that women be observed from the beginning to the end of their reproductive spans, entailing over 30 years of observations. Researchers more commonly compute cohort ASFRs from post-reproductive women retrospectively reporting their births. In these instances the cohort TFR is the same as the completed family size (CFS), where the CFS is the average number of live births reported by women who have survived past menopause. Even if women accurately report all their births, estimates of past fertility based on retrospective reports may differ from rates based on observed births (i.e. births recorded in a longitudinal study). Women who die may have different fertility from women who survive. We examine ways in which our rates may be biased in these ways later in this chapter.

Herero fertility by period

To examine temporal trends in Herero fertility, we computed age-specific fertility rates (ASFRs) for four periods from the 611 reproductive histories we collected in 1987–9. They are listed in Table 5.1. The number of births to women and the number of person years that women spent at risk of having a birth at each age during each period are given in the tables. The table also shows the total fertility rate for each period (the period TFR) corresponding to each set of period ASFRs. We smoothed irregularities in the ASFRs caused by small sample sizes by collapsing the data into 5-year age classes. We adjusted the TFRs by multiplying the sum of the ASFRs by the width of the age-classes. Altogether, there were 12 774 person years and 1921 births in 1909 through 1986.

We computed the fertility rates for three sequential 10-year periods and for the period 1909–56 to illustrate the transition from very low to very high fertility rates among Herero women. The first period begins in 1909 because that is the year that the oldest woman we met became 15. The last period ends the year before we began this study. We combined the fertility rates of women reproducing in 1909–56 because of data sparseness.

Table 5.1. Age-specific fertility rates (ASFRs) by period, 1909–86. TFR is the total fertility rate

Period	Age class	No. births	Person years	ASFR
1909–1956	15–19	151	1146	0.132
	20–24	161	932	0.173
	25–29	83	752	0.110
	30–34	27	590	0.046
	35–39	16	373	0.043
	40–44	5	190	0.026
	45–49	0	73	0.000
TFR				2.65
1957–1966	15–18	75	427	0.176
	20–24	83	412	0.201
	25–29	71	386	0.184
	30–34	36	335	0.107
	35–39	27	370	0.073
	40–44	16	395	0.041
	45–49	4	297	0.013
TFR				3.98
1967–1976	15–19	86	447	0.192
	20–24	114	399	0.286
	25–29	96	422	0.227
	30–34	71	394	0.180
	35–39	43	373	0.115
	40–44	22	323	0.068
	45–49	5	367	0.014
TFR				5.41
1977–1986	15–19	156	713	0.219
	20–24	224	644	0.348
	25–29	132	441	0.299
	30–34	99	397	0.249
	35–39	81	422	0.192
	40–44	31	391	0.079
	45–49	6	363	0.017
TFR				7.02

There are fewer than 100 person years accrued before 1925, and there are no person years to estimate fertility for 45–9-year-old women until 1939. However, we computed fertility rates for three subperiods of 1909–56 for age-classes for which we have sufficient data, shown in Table 5.2; it appears that fertility of Herero women was uniformly low throughout 1909–56.

Fig. 5.1 clearly illustrates a dramatic increase in Herero fertility rates.

Table 5.2.   Age-specific fertility rates (ASFRs) by period, 1909–56. TFR is the total fertility rate

Period	Age class	No. births	Person years	ASFR
1909–1936	15–19	49	382	0.128
	20–24	35	200	0.175
	25–29	9	77	0.117
1937–1946	15–19	52	371	0.140
	20–24	68	395	0.172
	25–29	34	304	0.112
	30–34	4	156	0.026
1947–1956	15–19	50	393	0.127
	20–24	58	337	0.172
	25–29	40	371	0.108
	30–34	23	395	0.058
	35–39	14	300	0.047
	40–44	2	151	0.013
	45–49	0	60	0.000
TFR				2.63

This figure is a plot of the fertility rates in Table 5.1. The curves for the different time periods show that fertility was lowest in the period 1909–56, during which the TFR was only 2.65. Fertility began increasing among women of all ages in the period 1957–66, resulting in a TFR of 7.02 for the most recent period, 1977–86. This increase in fertility is unusually dramatic but reflects true trends in the data.

Each period shows the age pattern of fertility typical of natural fertility populations in which marital fertility rates peak in the mid-20s and decline from then on (Henry 1961; Wood 1989). We combined married and unmarried women in our estimates because marriage is not a strong predictor of Herero fertility (see Chapter 7).

Our estimates of Herero fertility are comparable to previous estimates of their fertility and to overall levels of fertility in Botswana. In the 1970s, Almagor (1982a) estimated that the Herero had a TFR of 6.45.[1] This value is intermediate and therefore consistent with the rates we report for 1967–76 and 1977–86. Our estimate of recent Herero fertility is slightly higher than levels reported throughout Botswana earlier in the decade. The total fertility rate of rural women in Botswana in 1981 was 6.65, about half a birth higher than the average TFR among all women in Botswana in 1981 (Central Statistics Office 1987). The 1984 *Botswana family health survey* (Manyeneng *et al.* 1985) estimated the overall total fertility rate to be

---

[1] Almagor (1982a) sampled 106 Mbanderu women living in the Lake Ngami area.

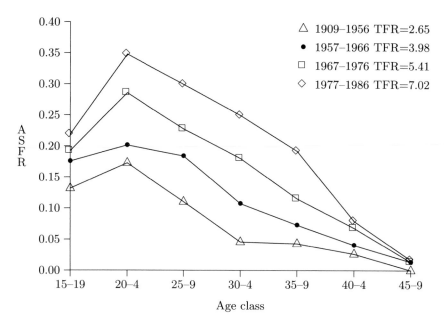

Fig. 5.1. Herero age-specific fertility rates (ASFRs) for four periods. TFR is the total fertility rate.

6.46. The fertility rates from the Botswana census and the FHS may be lower than our Herero rates because of differences in the timing of the surveys, because of regional variation in fertility in Botswana, or because of sampling error. If the 1981 census, the 1984 FHS, and our survey are all accurate, then fertility has been increasing in Botswana in the 1980s. It is also possible that women living in Ngamiland have higher fertility than most rural women in Botswana.

However, as a region, Ngamiland appears to have a history of lower fertility than the rest of Botswana. The TFR computed from the 1971 census for the whole country was 5.79 (Central Statistics Office 1972). At the same time, the TFR in Ngamiland was only 4.69. The completed family size (CFS) of women in Ngamiland also indicates that fertility was even lower in the past. Women aged 45–9 and 50+ reported having had an average of only 4.00 and 3.75 live births, respectively, in their lifetime. Again, these rates were among the lowest reported in the various regions of Botswana in 1971.

Similarly, Nancy Howell estimated that the CFS of !Kung women who were post-reproductive in 1968 was 4.69 (Howell 1979). Howell also examined the CFS of cohorts of these women and found that older women had higher fertility than younger women, indicating that !Kung fertility had been declining in the first half of the century. The !Kung TFR during the period 1963–73 was 4.28, slightly lower than the fertility rate of the older, post-reproductive women. The !Kung reside among Herero throughout many areas of Ngamiland. Although the reproductive rates recorded by Nancy Howell appeared unusually low at the time, the !Kung actually had higher fertility than the Herero and other peoples in the region. Harpending and Draper (1990) argued that !Kung fertility declined in the 1950s in response to accelerating contact with Bantu people, among whom sexually-transmitted diseases were rife. In Chapter 9, we contrast !Kung and Herero demographic rates and describe this more explicitly.

TFRs as low as the Herero's are not unknown in Africa. Caldwell and Caldwell (1983) thoroughly summarized the range of TFRs reported in Africa. They noted TFRs lower than 4.00 in many parts of Zaire, Gabon, Cameroon, Niger, and the Central African Republic during the late 1950s and early 1960s. They found TFRs of 4.00–5.00 documented in other parts of Zaire, Cameroon, the Central African Republic, and in parts of Sierra Leone and the Sudan during the same period. Eastern Zaire had an overall TFR of 2.8 in the late 1950s. Other sources have reported similarly low levels of fertility. TFRs of 2.13 and 2.64 were estimated for two regions of the Congo in 1955–7 (Romaniuk 1968a).

There are few sources with estimates of fertility in Africa before 1955, when Herero fertility was at its minimum, so it is not surprising that the Herero rates are among the lowest reported. The causes of low fertility in these regions appear to be related to STDs, which became easier to control following the advent of penicillin in the 1940s (see following chapter).

Sources of data bias

When estimates of fertility are based on retrospective reports, we must consider the possibility that estimates are biased by misreporting of births or selective maternal mortality. Demographers are leery of accepting demographic rates based on retrospective reports because older women tend to report fewer births than expected from estimates of current fertility rates. As a result, demographers often attribute apparent increases in fertility to old women failing to report all their births. There is also concern that the fertility of women who have survived to report their births may not be representative of all women born in the past. Higher mortality among women who had the most births may cause past fertility to be under-estimated.

Under-reporting of births

Under-reported births in fertility histories may be due to old women omitting children because the children died or because the children were born so long ago that they have been forgotten. Older women usually have more deceased children than younger women so their fertility may appear to be lower because they did not report all their deceased children. Demographers also attribute shortfalls in births to 'memory lapse' in old women. Brittain (1991), who found little evidence of reporting errors due to memory loss in the East Carribean, suggested that evidence for memory loss in other studies (i.e. Blacker and Brass 1979) may be due to cultural misunderstandings in questionnaires, such as insensitivity to taboos on speaking of the dead. From our point of view, it is hard to believe that women can 'forget' births, but it is certainly understandable that women would rather not talk about deceased loved ones.

Several lines of evidence indicate that our estimates of Herero fertility are not biased by older women under-reporting deceased offspring or 'forgetting' about births that they had long ago. First, older women report higher mortality among their infants and toddlers than younger women. During the period of fertility increase, infant mortality has *decreased* from 128 per 1000 live births to 63. Mortality from age 1 through 4 has also decreased from 87 per 1000 to 31 (see Chapter 3). This means that under-reporting of deaths cannot account for the low fertility we observed. There is also no indication that we have grossly under-estimated past offspring mortality. Our estimate of infant mortality was 117 per 1000 in 1960–74 while the 1971 Botswana census estimate was 97 per 1000 (Central Statistics Office 1972; Finch and Way 1981). Our higher Herero mortality rate is probably due to higher overall levels of mortality in Ngamiland (Central Statistics Office 1972).

Second, if old women under-report births because they are forgetful, births they had at younger ages should be under-reported more than births they had at older ages. Children born longest ago were born earliest in their mothers' reproductive spans so they are the most likely to be forgotten. In our data the opposite pattern appears—the largest deficit of births occurs at the end of the reproductive span. Regardless of when women were born, they report having their first births at the same ages. As they age, they report having fewer and fewer births. We show analytically in Chapter 10 that the mean age of child-bearing during the two earliest periods was about 22 years. Following the increase in fertility, the mean age of child-bearing increased to about 29 years. The unusually low mean of 22 years indicates that reproduction was concentrated at early ages during 1909–66 and that many women experienced truncated reproductive spans.

Table 5.3, which shows the mean age at first birth and the mean age at last birth for post-reproductive women born in three periods, also shows this trend. The average age that women report having their first birth is about 20, and there is very little variability among the cohorts. In contrast, there is nearly a 5-year increase in the average age at which women cease reproduction between the oldest and youngest cohorts. It also appears that the primary sterility rate (the percentage of women never having a

Table 5.3. Mean age at first and last birth of post-reproductive women by cohort

Birth cohort	n	No. sterile	First birth	SE	Last birth	SE
1894–1921	92	11	19.65	0.49	26.91	0.92
1922–1931	65	9	19.59	0.67	29.77	1.30
1932–1941	82	14	19.59	0.42	32.41	1.22

live birth) increased from 12 per cent to 17 per cent. In Chapter 9 we use survival analysis to compare the ages at which two groups of Herero women had their first birth and found no temporal change.

The deficit of births at the end rather than at the beginning of the reproductive span also supports our assertion that our fertility rates are not seriously biased by under-reporting of deceased offspring. Children born to women early in in the reproductive span are older and therefore more likely to be deceased than children born more recently, yet these are precisely the births being reported.

The secondary sex ratio (the sex ratio among new-borns) is also near unity. In parts of the world where there are strong sex preferences for children that lead to high sex differentials in mortality, there is a tendency to report fewer births of the less desired sex. Although we have observed an extremely high male mortality rate among the Herero, the sex ratio at birth since 1960 is 1.05 and not significantly different from 1. Before 1960, when female mortality was higher, though not significantly so, the sex ratio at birth was 1.13 but, also, was not significantly different from one. This means that Herero are not preferentially reporting births of one sex more than the other.

The shape of the Herero population pyramid shown in Chapter 2 shows patterns typical of a population that has undergone a fertility transition. The base of the pyramid is broad, like that of a population with a high birth-rate. The upper portion of the pyramid, however, is narrow rather than tapered, indicating that fertility was lower in the past.

Selective maternal mortality

In subsequent sections we estimate family size distributions for various cohorts of post-reproductive women. These distributions are calculated from information obtained from women who themselves survived to the end of the reproductive period. There may be bias in information collected this way since child-bearing itself may be an important cause of mortality of women during the reproductive years. In this case the women who survived to be interviewed may be a less fertile subset of the cohort that began reproduction with them. Our retrospective interview information may under-estimate true fertility rates. In this section we construct several models of maternal mortality using probability distributions commonly used to approximate the distribution of family sizes in human populations. We show that bias arising from maternal mortality is not very large or significant.

We assume that in the absence of any maternal mortality the distribution of family sizes among post-menopausal women would conform to one of several parametric distributions. We will discuss the cases of Poisson, negative binomial and modified geometric distributions. We choose the Poisson and negative binomial distributions because they have properties desirable for examining biological properties of fertility and have been used by other researchers (Brass 1958; Cavalli-Sforza and Bodmer 1971; Howell 1979; Golbeck 1981). The geometric distribution is appropriate for modelling family size distributions in populations where the probability of becoming sterile after each birth is constant. We develop a modified geometric distribution with parameters related to the primary and secondary sterility rates in the population.

We also assume that the rate of maternal mortality is a constant μ per confinement. That is, a fraction $1 - \mu$ of women survive the birth of each child while a fraction μ die. Since the rate is constant per confinement, the fraction of a cohort who survive the birth of the kth child is $(1 - \mu)^k$. For example, if a number n_5 of a cohort of women entering child-bearing were to have exactly five births with no maternal mortality, we would observe only $n_5(1 - \mu)^5$ at the end of child-bearing because of maternal mortality. If maternal mortality were as high as 5 per cent per confinement ($\mu = 0.05$) and if 100 were to have no children at the end of child-bearing while another 100 were to have five births in the absence of death associated with childbirth, we would observe 100 childless women when we interviewed in the population but only 77 women (100×0.95^5) who had had five births.

Empirical evidence suggests that the true pattern of maternal mortality is J-shaped, being highest at the first and also at the higher ordered parities (Heady and Daly 1955; Yerushalmy et al. 1956; Nortman 1974). Women with high parity may also have reduced life-spans beyond the reproductive years. Although these factors imply an accelerating rate of maternal mortality, because only a proportion of women who reproduce have subsequent births the additional bias introduced may not be large.

Poisson distribution   A simple model of the distribution of family sizes is the Poisson distribution, which would arise if the hazard of giving birth were constant among all women during the child-bearing years. In this case the distribution of family sizes p_x would follow

$$p_x = \frac{e^{-\lambda}\lambda^x}{x!} \qquad x = 0, 1, \ldots$$

in the absence of maternal mortality. The mean and the variance of this distribution are both equal to λ. Note that the mean of the family size distribution is the same as the completed family size (CFS).

With maternal deaths occurring at a rate of μ per confinement, the frequency of post-menopausal women who had had x births would be proportional to

$$f_x = \frac{e^{-\lambda}\lambda^x}{x!}(1-\mu)^x \qquad x = 0, 1, \ldots$$

In order to derive the probability distribution of observed family sizes each f_x must be divided by the sum of all the f's. Since

$$\sum_{i=0}^{\infty}\frac{e^{-\lambda}\lambda^x}{x!}(1-\mu)^x = e^{-\lambda\mu}$$

the probability distribution of family size as modified by the occurrence of maternal mortality is

$$p_x = \frac{e^{-\lambda(1-\mu)}\lambda(1-\mu)^x}{x!} \qquad x = 0, 1, \ldots$$

This is again a Poisson distribution with parameter $\lambda(1-\mu)$. The family sizes observed at the end of child-bearing would be reduced by maternal mortality by $1-\mu$, that is by one less the proportion of women who die *per confinement*. A high rate of maternal mortality would be about 1 per cent per confinement (Royston and Lopez 1987), causing a 1 per cent change in the estimate of CFS. This is such a small change that it is of a lower order of magnitude than our sampling error.

There are several other probability distributions that are reasonable candidates for modelling the distribution of family sizes.

Negative binomial distribution   Several processes might lead to a negative binomial distribution of family sizes. For example, if births occurred to each woman according to a Poisson process while the intensity of the process, i.e. the intrinsic fecundity of the woman, varied according to a gamma distribution, the population distribution would be negative binomial. The distribution is

$$p_x = \binom{x+r-1}{x}p^r q^x \qquad x = 0, 1, \ldots, \; r > 0, \; 0 \le p \le 1, \; q = 1-p.$$

The mean of this distribution is rq/p and the variance is rq/p^2. If maternal mortality occurs at rate μ per confinement, the distribution of family sizes observed at the end of reproduction becomes

$$p_x = \binom{x+r-1}{x}(p+q\mu)^r(q-q\mu)^x \qquad x = 0, 1, \ldots$$

This is again a negative binomial distribution with the same parameter r as the original but with the second parameter changed to $p+q\mu$. The mean is now $r(q - q\mu)/(p + q\mu)$. The effect of maternal mortality is to change the observed mean (the CFS) by the rate of maternal mortality, just as in the case of the Poisson distribution.

Modified geometric A geometric distribution of family size would result if a cohort of women experienced a constant parity progression ratio (PPR). That is, from a process in which the probability that women who have an nth birth have an $n + 1$th birth, $n = 0\ldots$, is constant across all n. A model that specifies that the PPR from 0 to 1 births is 0.85 and that each later PPR is 0.75 fits the family size distribution of Herero women past menopause remarkably well. This model leads to a modified geometric distribution of family size since the 0-category is specified separately. If π_0 is the primary sterility rate (in our case, 0.15) and if π is the probability of terminating reproduction after any order birth, the resulting distribution of family sizes is

$$\begin{aligned} p_0 &= \pi_0 \\ p_x &= (1 - \pi_0)(1 - \pi)^{i-1}\pi \qquad x = 1, 2, \ldots \end{aligned}$$

The mean of this distribution is $(1 - \pi_0)/\pi$. Using our simple representation of Herero PPRs this becomes $0.85/0.25 = 3.4$.

If this distribution is modified by allowing a constant probability μ of maternal mortality per birth the new distribution is again a modified geometric

$$\begin{aligned} p_0 &= \pi_0' \\ p_x &= (1 - \pi_0')(1 - \pi')^{i-1}\pi' \qquad x = 1, 2, \ldots \end{aligned}$$

with

$$\begin{aligned} \pi_0' &= \frac{\pi_0(\pi + (1 - \pi)\mu)}{\mu\pi_0 + \pi(1 - \mu)} \\ \pi' &= \pi + (1 - \pi)\mu. \end{aligned}$$

Using our estimates $\pi_0 = 0.15$ and $\pi = 0.25$ that fit the Herero data (see below), we can compute that a maternal mortality rate of 1 per cent per birth would reduce the observed CFS from 3.4 to 3.28, i.e. a change of less than 4 per cent.

These models show that even a rate of maternal mortality as high as 1 per cent does not lead to a serious bias when we estimate CFS from retrospective fertility histories. We have only solved several special cases here, and it is probably possible to construct feasible models where the bias is large. On the other hand the modified geometric model is an excellent fit to the Herero data so that a radically different model would not be like the real structure of the Herero family size distribution.

Family size distribution

Direct

Estimates of overall fertility

Period ASFRs capture changes in fertility as women age as well as changes in fertility through time. TFRs computed from ASFRs are also useful for summarizing differences in fertility between populations. However, unless fertility is constant, period rates are not appropriate summaries of the fertility of cohorts of women. For example, women aged 40–4 in the period 1977–86 were born in 1932–46; these women were 15–19 in 1947–65. Thus, none of the TFRs we calculated refers to the experience of a single birth cohort of Herero women. Rather, each TFR encapsulates the fertility experience of women born in four different decades, during which time fertility has undergone a dramatic transition.

In contrast, the completed family size (CFS), which is the mean number of live births born to women aged past menopause, describes the experience of a defined group of women, although it reveals nothing about the timing of reproduction. The CFS is often the only measure of fertility appropriate for making comparisons among small populations. It has few data requirements so it can be accurately calculated in populations where women cannot report their ages but can report whether they have reached menopause, and where there are too few data from which to reliably estimate ASFRs.

The CFS is a function of the distribution of family sizes in a population. Fig. 5.2 shows the frequency of family sizes among the 239 post-reproductive Herero women (those aged 45 years or more in 1986) whom we met. Apparently most women had small families—about 15 per cent had no births and more than half had two or fewer. Family sizes of only one are the most frequent. A secondary peak at parity six hints at bimodality. The CFS of these women is 3.47, which is quite low. CFSs less than five in natural fertility populations are often associated with unusual circumstances, such as sterilizing diseases or sub-fecundity.

The national population of Botswana does not show similarly low rates

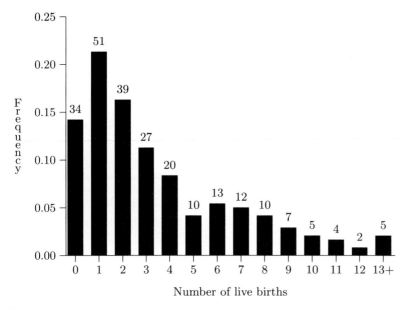

Fig. 5.2.   The distribution of completed family sizes among Herero women.

of fertility. In 1981, the Botswana census found that women older than age 45 reported having had an average of 5.93 live births (Central Statistics Office 1981). Among women aged 45–9, the CFS was 6.42, comparable to the CFS of 6.84 found among 45–9 year old women by the 1984 *Family health survey* (Manyeneng *et al.* 1985). However, the 1971 Botswana census recorded below average fertility among women in Ngamiland (see above). The TFR was only 4.69 in 1971, and women 45–9 years old had had only 4.00 births. Almagor (1982*a*) also found that 11 Mbanderu women aged 45–9 in his study in the 1970s had an average of only 5.18 births.

Few data on fertility of other African pastoralists are available for comparison. Among nomadic and sedentary Baggara cattle pastoralists in the Sudan, CFSs were 4.6 and 5.5, respectively (Henin 1968). Interestingly, Henin cites higher childlessness rates and higher prevalences of STDs among the nomadic group, indicating that STDs may also be responsible for fertility differentials among them. In the Sahel, nomadic Tamasheq and Fulani pastoralists had CFSs ranging from 4.6 to 7.1 (Hill *et al.* 1983). Another group of Turkana women who had spent their reproductive years as nomadic pastoralists had 7.32 births (Brainard 1986).

The !Kung Bushmen, Khoisan hunter-gatherers residing in the same region as Herero, have one of the lowest CFSs in Africa. In the 1960s, the !Kung CFS was estimated at 4.7 (Howell 1979) and 4.0 (Harpending

Table 5.4. Number of births to post-reproductive Herero women by cohort

Birth cohort	No. women	No. births	Mean	SE
1894–1921	92	241	2.62	0.25
1922–1931	65	227	3.49	0.39
1932–1941	82	362	4.41	0.44

and Wandsnider 1982). Outside Africa, CFSs as low as those found among Herero have been noted in horticultural foraging populations such as the Cayapo Indians of Brazil (Salzano 1971) and the Kiunga of Papua New Guinea (Serjeantson 1975), who had CFSs of 3.8 and 3.4, respectively. Campbell and Wood (1988) surveyed the fertility of other small populations.

Bongaarts and Potter (1983) estimated that primary sterility rates of about 3–5 per cent can be expected in populations that do not rely on contraceptives and that have normal levels of fertility. The childlessness rate of 15 per cent among post-reproductive Herero women places them well beyond the range considered normal. However, given the overall levels of fertility, this childlessness rate is relatively low. In the Congo, childlessness rates as high as 40 per cent have been recorded (Romaniuk 1968a). Romaniuk (1968b) and Frank (1983) recorded similarly high levels of primary sterility.

Differences by cohorts

Although useful for comparisons, the Herero CFS is a summary of the reproductive performance of women who were born in a nearly 50-year time span, from 1894 to 1941, concealing any heterogeneity among women born in various years. To test for temporal trends in fertility, we grouped the data into three birth cohorts, 1894–1921, 1922–31 and 1932–41. Table 5.4 shows the numbers of women born in these cohorts and their total numbers of live births. The oldest cohort of women, those born in 1894–1921, have the lowest CFS (2.62), while the youngest cohort has the highest (4.41). The cohort of women born in 1922–31 is intermediate with a CFS of 3.49. Using the F-test to compare the between mean variability (s_B^2) with the within-group variability (s_W^2) (Anderson *et al.* 1981), the probability that all three means are equal is less than 1 in 100 ($s_B^2/s_W^2 = 6.57$, 2, 230 d.f.). It appears that the older women had much lower fertility than the younger women in this sample.

Table 5.5. Observed and weighted family size distributions of informants' mothers. Data come from offspring reporting their mothers' fertility

Family size	Observed no.	Weighted no.
1	4	4.00
2	7	3.50
3	6	2.00
4	8	2.00
5	8	1.60
6	12	2.00
7	9	1.29
8	6	0.75
9	2	0.22
10	4	0.40
11	2	0.18
12	0	0.00
13	2	0.15

Indirect

Seventy informants whose mothers were either post-reproductive or post-reproductive at the time of their death were asked how many births their mothers had had. A list of the number of mothers with various family sizes is given in Table 5.5. We used this information to compute indirect estimates of completed fertility and the frequency of family sizes using the technique described by Harpending and Draper (1990). We use these estimates to cross-check our directly obtained estimates and to make inferences about fertility further into the past.

We simply asked informants to name their living maternal siblings and to tell us how many others had died. Since members of large sibships have a greater chance of being ascertained than members of smaller sibships, we must weight their responses before using them to estimate fertility. For example, assuming that mortality is independent of sibship size, individuals whose mothers had ten births are ten times more likely to be ascertained than individuals whose mothers had only one birth. Harpending and Draper (1990) describe a method for weighting each observation such that, if n_i is the number of informants with sibships of size $i, i = 1, 2, 3, \ldots, k$, where k is the maximum family size, then the imputed number of mothers m_i can be estimated by

$$m_i = \frac{n_i}{i}.$$

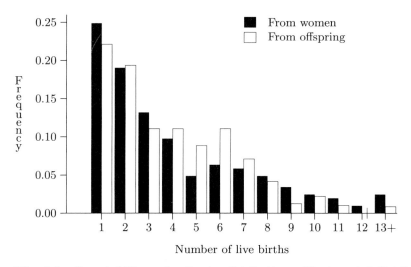

Fig. 5.3. Imputed Herero family size distributions. The imputed distribution was estimated from offspring reporting their mothers' fertility. The distribution of family sizes obtained directly from women we interviewed is shown for comparison.

The estimated frequency of each sibship size ($i > 0$) is thus

$$f_i = \frac{m_i}{\sum_j m_j}.$$

The estimated CFS of women having at least one live birth is then

$$\hat{\mu} = \sum ii f_i = \frac{\sum_i n_i}{\sum_i m_i}.$$

The resulting imputed number of mothers having various family sizes is given in Table 5.5. We used these data to generate the imputed (indirect) family size distribution in Figtre 5.3, which shows for comparison the directly obtained family size distribution in Fig. 5.2. The indirect estimate closely approximates that of the direct estimate and includes the secondary peak at parity six. The CFSs of women having at least one live birth are also similar, $\hat{\mu} = 3.9$ for the indirect estimate and 4.0 for the direct estimate.

The main purpose of indirectly computing the average family size is that we can infer the fertility rates of Herero women who are older than women that we interviewed. The average birth year of the mothers of informants was 1907. The average year of birth of women that we interviewed was 1925, making them 18 years younger on average than the mothers. Fertility is of considerable interest among Herero, and informants responded

Table 5.6. Observed and weighted familiy size distributions of the mothers of informants by cohort. Data come from offspring reporting their mothers' fertility

| | Mothers born 1870–1906 | | Mothers born 1907–1941 | |
Family size	Observed no.	Weighted no.	Observed no.	Weighted no.
1	0	0.00	4	4.00
2	4	2.00	3	1.50
3	2	0.67	4	1.33
4	3	0.75	5	1.25
5	6	1.20	2	0.40
6	8	1.33	4	0.67
7	5	0.71	4	0.57
8	3	0.38	3	0.38
9	2	0.22	0	0.00
10	2	0.20	2	0.20
11	0	0.00	2	0.18
12	0	0.00	0	0.00
13	0	0.00	2	1.15

with confidence when reporting their mothers' numbers of births. We have confidence in our indirect estimates because 14 of our informants supplied information about women who had been independently interviewed. In all 14 cases the answers matched exactly. Herero also are knowledgeable about their mothers' pregnancy wastage. Herero are more willing to discuss deceased siblings than deceased offspring.

Because the antiquity of low fertility among the Herero is of interest, we examined these data for temporal changes in fertility by partitioning the data into two maternal birth cohorts. We divided our sample at 1907 to divide the number of informants reporting on their mothers' fertility exactly in half. The observed and weighted numbers of family sizes by cohort are in Table 5.6. We computed the standard errors using the formula in Harpending and Draper (1990). The average family size of mothers who had at least one birth in the older cohort is 4.7 ± 0.70 compared to only 3.3 ± 0.35 in the younger cohort. The unweighted average birth year of mothers in each cohort was 1891 (ranging from 1870 to 1906) and 1922 (ranging from 1907 to 1941). On the average, the older mothers were born 29 years earlier. The indirect estimates of CFSs compare with means of 3.0, 4.0, and 5.3 for the direct estimates of women born in the periods 1894–1921, 1922–31, and 1932–41, respectively. It appears that fertility was higher among the older women, bottomed out in the early years of this century, and then increased again when antibiotics became available in rural Botswana.

If the trend in the data is genuine, then the cause of infertility had its greatest impact among women born in the two decades after the turn of the century. This implies that the cause of low fertility may have its roots early in this century. It is possible that the difference in fertility between the two cohorts of mothers is related to disruptions caused by the Herero–German War or to differences in life-styles in Namibia and Botswana. All but a few women in both cohorts, however, spent the majority of their child-bearing years in Botswana so that the potential effects of these factors are probably small in this sample of women.

Parity progression ratios

We used the directly and indirectly obtained family size distributions to compute parity progression ratios (PPRs). Each PPR $i, i = 0, 1, 2, \ldots, k - 1$, where k is the maximum family size, is the proportion of women who, having had an ith birth, have an $i + 1$th birth. Fig. 5.4 shows the two sets of PPRs. The PPR for $i = 0$ is about 0.85, indicating that about 85 per cent of all women had a first birth, or, conversely, that 15 per cent never had at least one birth. The rest of the PPRs are around 0.75, indicating that about 25 per cent of women become sterile after each birth until it is zero at the maximum family size. Since the number of women who had zero births cannot be estimated indirectly, the indirect PPRs start at $i = 1$. The PPRs from the indirect estimates are close at lower parities, suggesting similar patterns of fertility.

The shape of these curves also indicates something about the reproductive behaviour of Herero women. The overall shape of the curves is concave downwards, a shape characteristic of natural fertility populations (Howell 1979). The shape of PPR curves in contracepting populations tend to be concave upwards due to most women terminating reproduction at lower parities so that PPRs decline more rapidly. It is not surprising that the Herero PPRs are concave downwards since few Herero use contraceptives. We would be concerned about the quality of our data were this pattern absent. Characterizing the Herero as a natural fertility population is useful since we can assume that Herero do not deliberately limit their fertility (Henry 1961).

Summary and conclusions

The period TFR of Herero women reproducing in 1909–56 indicates that they have had abnormally low fertility since the beginning of this century. Fertility has been increasing among women of all age classes since the late 1950s. The TFR for the most recent period, 1977–86, is 7.02.

We also computed the CFSs for three cohorts of women born in 1894 through 1941. The oldest women had the lowest fertility. The CFS of all

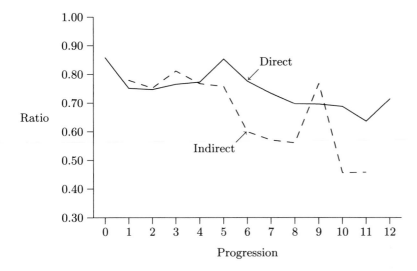

Fig. 5.4. Herero parity progression ratios. Direct is from interviewed women. Indirect is from offspring reporting their mothers' fertility.

women was 3.47. Our estimates of low fertility were confirmed by indirect estimates of the fertility of the mothers of our informants. The parity of the most recently born mothers of informants was nearly the same as the parity that we estimated from women that we interviewed. Informants whose mothers were born longer ago, however, had higher fertility.

We considered several sources of bias in our data and concluded that they were probably not substantial. We derived a model estimating the bias introduced by maternal mortality in retrospective fertility reports. The potential bias from this source is very small and is probably less worrisome than sampling error.

Altogether, these findings indicate that the Herero have been afflicted with pathologically low levels of fertility since the late nineteenth century. Fertility was apparently declining early in this century and remained low and unchanging during 1909–56. It has been increasing ever since.

A comparison of the Herero CFS with CFSs from the Botswana census and the 1984 *Family health survey* suggests that Herero fertility was unusually low. A comparison of Herero fertility with their !Kung neigbours and with other women in Ngamiland, however, shows that this region has a history of lower than average fertility. Historical accounts support our findings of abnormally low fertility. Steenkamp (1944) and Gibson (1959) addressed the possibility that the Herero were actually committing 'tribal suicide' by refusing to bear children.

General references to low fertility and concern with depopulation in

Botswana appear in other historical sources. Schapera (1947) investigated these rumours and, based on a crude estimate of the net reproduction rate of women living in the eastern part of the country, concluded that there was not a depopulation problem in Botswana. Nevertheless, fertility was low. Post-reproductive women reported having 2.54 daughters each. Assuming a sex ratio of 1.05 at birth, this means that women had only 5.21 births. More recently, high incidences of STDs were associated with lower fertility at Mahalapye (Edlinger 1988).

Interestingly, Adadevoh (1974) dismissed low fertility in Botswana as being due to emigration of males seeking employment in other areas. Unlike the Tswana, however, few Herero have worked in the South African mines. Because of sexual permissiveness in and out of marriage in Botswana, it is possible that spousal separation would have no effect on fertility. Demographers have also attributed low fertility rates to older women 'forgetting' that they gave birth to some of their children, especially if the children died young (Brass 1968). However, there is no evidence in these data suggesting that Herero under-report deceased or living children. We examine the causes and implications of low Herero fertility in the next chapter.

6
Causes of the fertility transition

Demographers have been aware of substantial fertility variation in African census and survey data for several decades. Coale (1968) observed a 'high fertility ridge' and a low fertility region in population data from the 1950s and early 1960s. Total fertility rates (TFRs) ranged from 3.5 to more than 8. Overall TFRs for the sub-Saharan countries that he included (which did not include Southern Africa) were 6.1–6.2. However, the distribution was patchy. Regions with very high fertility neigboured those with much lower fertility. Romaniuk (1968*b*) examined regional heterogeneity in national population data. Both Romaniuk (1968*b*) and Adadevoh (1974) considered correlates of low fertility, such as certain marriage patterns, induced abortion, contraception, malnutrition, and diseases. They found sexually-transmitted diseases (STDs) to be outstanding correlates of sub-fertility. Frank (1983), Caldwell and Caldwell, (1983) and Doenges and Newman (1989) have reworked these data. All implicate STDs as important causes of low fertility. STDs have become a variable essential to understanding fertility differentials in African societies (Mammo and Morgan 1986).

Low fertility and high childlessness rates among post-reproductive Herero women suggest that they were affected by the same infectious agents afflicting other African populations. In the previous chapter, we showed that nearly 15 per cent of all post-reproductive women never had a live birth. Although higher primary sterility rates have been observed in other parts of Africa, our TFR estimate of 2.65 during the early part of this century is among the lowest on record. Herero experienced truncated reproductive spans so that over 50 per cent of women had two or fewer births. Through indirect estimates of the fertility of our informants' mothers, we confirmed that low Herero fertility predates the turn of the century. An increase in fertility in the period 1957–66 appears to be due to an increase in the ages at which women cease child-bearing. The increase in the total fertility rate for the period 1957–66 coincides with the appearance of mobile medical dispensaries in north-western Botswana (van Dam and Molosiwa 1987).

In addition to STDs, we consider below other possible causes of low fertility in Herero. Our goal is to find a cause with consequences so severe that it could cause the pathologically low levels of fertility that we recorded. The cause must have an epidemiology that would allow for the apparent increase in fertility at the appropriate time. We discuss the effects of a number of diseases on fertility. We also consider the possibility that ecological factors are responsible for variability in Herero reproductive rates. In particular, we examine the importance of breast-feeding patterns, health, and activity levels.

Diseases

Disease can affect fertility by causing sterility, by interfering with reproductive functioning or by contributing to pregnancy wastage. In addition to causing delay between live births, pregnancy wastage may also cause secondary infections that lead to sterility. McFalls and McFalls (1984) describe the effects of infections such as tuberculosis (TB), malaria, filariasis, schistosomiasis, and sexually-transmitted diseases (STDs) on fertility. Belsey (1976) has reviewed their epidemiology in sub-Saharan Africa. Among these diseases, syphilis and pelvic inflammatory disease (PID) resulting from gonococcal, chlamydial, and other lower genital tract infections are the major correlates of low fertility in sub-Saharan Africa (Belsey 1976; Muir and Belsey 1980; Frank 1983; Caldwell and Caldwell 1983; Mabey *et al.* 1985; Cates *et al.* 1988). Other infections appear to have either smaller effects on fertility, have a low known incidence in sub-Saharan Africa (McFalls and McFalls 1984; Belsey 1976), or have been ignored in studies of sub-fertility (McFalls and McFalls 1984). Below we consider the potential effects of those diseases occurring in Botswana on fertility and discuss their correspondence to the pattern of Herero fertility.

Tuberculosis

Genital TB occurs when the bacillus *Mycobacterium tuberculosis* (though sometimes *Mycobacterium bovis* or other bacteria are involved) spreads from its site of primary infection (the lung in the case of *M. tuberculosis*) through the lymph and vascular systems into the reproductive organs (McFalls and McFalls 1984). Sterility in females results from the bilateral formation of tubercles in the Fallopian tubes. These tubercles may impede movement of germ cells through the tubes making conception and implantation improbable. In severe cases, genital TB causes total tubal closure. Since genital TB is frequently symptomless, the proportion of TB cases that affects the genitals is unknown. Most estimates are based on the proportion of women with genital TB who appear at infertility clinics so that the prevalence in the general population is unknown. Additionally, the time-scale necessary for TB to progress to genital infection and cause sterility has not been established. However, some researchers have argued that genital TB may have a significant impact on reproductive performance. McFalls and McFalls (1984), for example, are convinced that genital TB was largely responsible for low fertility among Black Americans earlier in this century. Others (Farley 1970; Wright and Pirie 1984; Tolnay 1989) have blamed STDs.

In any case, TB affects only a fraction of women before and during their reproductive years. In turn, only a fraction of these cases affects the genitals so the incidence of TB must be high for the genital form to effect fertility at a population level. Although TB has been endemic in Botswana for many years, its antiquity is unknown. The prevalence of the disease among Herero is also unknown. In Ngamiland, TB is the major cause of institutional deaths (those in hospitals and other health clinics), although many children are now inoculated with the BCG vaccine (Ministry of Health 1982).

Twenty years ago, TB was quite prevalent among !Kung (Truswell and Hansen 1976). Howell (1979, p. 63) found that 56 per cent of !Kung tested positive for TB infection. She believed that TB was a major cause of death among !Kung. However, during field-work among the same !Kung population in Ngamiland, one of us (Harpending) found a lower frequency of !Kung testing positive for TB, although TB was common among the !Kung living in Ghanzi. Due to their higher standard of living, infection rates of Herero are probably much less than those of the impoverished !Kung. During the field-work for this study, we heard of only a few Herero who had been afflicted with TB in the past. In Namibia, O'Keefe and colleagues (1988) found that just under 70 per cent of !Kung patients had TB infections, compared to less that 10 per cent among Herero. Many !Kung live among Herero, who employ them as cattlehands.

In sum, it is unlikely that the frequency of TB among Herero is high enough to explain much of the low fertility. Moreover, high rates of TB infection reported among the !Kung coincide with increases, rather than decreases, in fertility among Herero, and TB is still endemic. Also, TB is not generally responsive to health post treatments so there is no obvious mechanism through which TB could decrease and lead to rising fertility rates.

Malaria

High fevers and anaemia caused by cell destruction from malaria may induce pregnancy wastage. Malaria has been prevalent in north-western Botswana for centuries; Andersson (1987) noted it there during his nineteenth century travels. However, malaria probably has had negligible measurable effects on fertility among Herero for several reasons. First, most are only sporadically exposed to infection. The *Anopheles* mosquito that transmits infection to humans reproduces in pools of standing water. Herero live in the semi-desert environment west of the Okavango Delta. The environment favourable to mosquito production occurs only during the rainy season so that mosquito concentrations are high for only a few months per year. Given the wide variability in annual rainfall in this area, risk of malarial infection varies considerably year to year. The mosquito breeding season is also truncated because the coldest part of the year follows the rainy season, and cold is non-conducive to mosquito reproduction. On the other hand, mosquitos are more likely to persist in areas along the Okavango Delta. The annual flooding of the Delta occasionally fills the ephemeral Lake Ngami. Since the Mbanderu heartland is Lake Ngami, the risk of malaria infection among Herero may vary geographically.

While the potential for pregnancy loss lengthening birth intervals among Herero exists, malaria has persisted throughout the decades in which fertility has been increasing. Also, given its seasonal occurrence in Botswana, only a small fraction of women would be at risk during a given outbreak. The Herero also appear to have more resistance to malaria than their !Kung neigbours. In March 1988, malaria was endemic among Herero and !Kung in the Dobe and Magopa areas of our study. Many more !Kung than Herero came to our camp seeking treatment for malaria. Communication with the local dispensary indicates that Herero did not preferentially seek treatment from the area medical clinic instead. It may be that the Herero style of dress affords them better protection against mosquito bites. Most women of reproductive age wear full-length nineteenth century style dresses, underlayered with at least three petticoats. On the other hand, clothing may not explain variation in risk of malaria since men and children in the two groups do not contrast as sharply in their dress.

Schistosomiasis

The impact of schistosomiasis on fertility is not clear. Worm infection results from skin penetration of waterborne *Schistosoma* larvae, which undergo a portion of their life cycle in certain freshwater snails. Schistosomiasis may affect fertility by producing lesions in genital tissues. An autopsy study in Zimbabwe by Gelfand and colleagues (1971) is one of the best-known studies of the effects of *Schistosoma* on the genital tract. They found that 50 per cent of women had lesions in pelvic organs, most commonly the Fallopian tubes (Gelfand *et al.* 1971). McFalls and McFalls (1984) believe that schistosomiasis probably has little effect on fecundity at the population level. They argue that most lesions found on reproductive organs are not severe enough to impair reproductive function. However, Bullough (1976) found that women suffering from either primary or secondary sterility had *S. haematobium* infection rates of about twice those of control women. While the actual lesions may have a minimal effect on reproductive performance, these findings suggest that schistosomiasis may promote secondary infection of the Fallopian tubes, although schistosomal salpingitis is not unknown either.

In any case, *Schistosoma* infection is rare or unknown among Herero. Howell (1979, p. 65) reported that this disease is unusual among the Herero's !Kung neigbours in the Dobe region, where there are no permanent freshwater sources other than wells. *Schistosoma* have infested the Okavango Delta, especially in Maun. Since Herero live away from the Delta, risk of infection from this source is low. Furthermore, Geldenhuys and Hallet (1967) found the prevalence of schistosomiasis to be relatively rare among all peoples of the Kalahari. Consequently, it cannot account for the low levels of fertility observed among Herero.

Sexually-transmitted diseases

Pelvic inflammatory disease

Pelvic inflammatory disease (PID) generally refers to the occurrence of salpingitis. It is often diagnosed in women reporting lower abdominal pain in association with cervical, uterine, and adnexal tenderness (Cates *et al.* 1988). Women suffering from PID have erythema, edema, and pus or exudate in the Fallopian tubes (Jacobson and Weström 1969). The majority of cases of PID in sub-Saharan Africa are attributed to *Chlamydia trachomatis* and *Neisseria gonorrhoea* (Belsey 1976; Mabey *et al.* 1985; Cates *et al.* 1987). Other bacteria have been implicated as well, but the possibility that these are secondary infections of *C. trachomatis* or *N. gonorrhoea* has not been ruled out.

C. *trachomatis* and *N. gonorrhoea* cause PID by ascending from the lower genital to upper genital tract through the cervix. The disease is self-limiting, but damage to the reproductive tract results from scarring of one or both Fallopian tubes during post-infection healing. These scars can impede tubal motility or damage tubal mucosa and cilia, thereby interfering with the movement of gametes through the reproductive tract and reducing the likelihood of fertilization. These same factors impede the transfer of zygotes to the uterus and increase the probability of ecoptic pregnancy in women with PID (Muir and Belsey 1980). Tubal occlusion can result from a single PID episode with the risk of occlusion increasing with repeated infection. Although infection can occur in only one Fallopian tube, bilateral infection is normal so that bilateral occlusion and infertility appear to be the ultimate outcome of repeated infection. Some evidence indicates that PID may cause ovarian failure such as through thickening of the ovarian capsule, thereby preventing release of ova (McFalls and McFalls 1984). Although the fertility prognosis of PID episodes is good for early treatment, once scarring or occlusion has occurred pharmacological treatment of PID apparently does not improve reproductive performance.

The frequencies of *C. trachomatis* and *N. gonorrhoea* PID episodes are highest at the beginning of the menstrual cycle (Cates *et al.* 1988). The biotic environment of the lower genital tract early in the cycle may favour proliferation of unfavourable organisms. The loss of the cervical mucus plug during menses may enhance the chances that they enter the upper reproductive tract. The plug may act as a barrier against disease. The flux of menstrual blood through the Fallopian tubes and the greater vulnerability of tissue exposed by the sloughing of the endometrium may also increase the opportunity for infection. Consequently, variation in the length of menses and the frequency of cycles may be important correlates of PID risk among individuals and populations in which these factors vary. Thus, populations characterized by later sexual maturity and prolonged postpartum amenorrhoea may also be characterized by a lower incidence of PID than populations where menses and sexual activity follow parturition more quickly. Since women are amenorrhoeic during pregnancy, pregnancy would seemingly provide an additional protective component against PID. Several studies show, however, that many women who have chlamydial or gonorrhoeal infections when they give birth experience PID episodes postpartum.

Syphilis

The effects of syphilis on fertility in sub-Saharan Africa have received less attention. Syphilis causes pregnancy wastage rather than sterility. With respect to fertility, it is largely a self-limiting disease. The disease is caused by *Treponema pallidum*. Fetuses of women afflicted with primary or secondary syphilis have a high chance of becoming infected. An infected fetus may be either aborted, born dead, or born alive with congenital syphilis. The outcome of pregnancy has been related to the stage of maternal infection. Infected mothers who conceive in the early stage of syphilis are most likely to abort their fetuses. The chances of bearing a live born child, either with or without congenital syphilis, increase with the duration of infection in the mother. Syphilis becomes latent in most women after about two years, after which the chances of bearing healthy children are quite good. Untreated primary or secondary syphilis tends to produce immunity to reinfection. Reinfection is most likely in individuals who receive early treatment, but the chances of reinfection diminish the later the treatment occurs. In sum, syphilis can be an important cause of pregnancy loss, but its effect is limited to only one or two pregnancy losses in most women.

Prevalence of STDs among Herero

History in Africa   Gonorrhoea, chlamydia, and syphilis are widespread throughout Africa. The infections are transmitted in the same way and prevalent in the same places so it is difficult to sort out the effects of one from another. Moreover, in Africa, both yaws and endemic syphilis are prevalent. These diseases are transmitted non-venereally but are caused by treponema either serologically or morphologically indistinguishable from *T. pallidum*. Measuring the prevalence of venereal syphilis where there is yaws or endemic syphilis is therefore difficult. All three (yaws, endemic syphilis, and venereal syphilis) cause cross-immunity, and since yaws and endemic syphilis are childhood diseases, venereal syphilis does not become prevalent in areas where the other treponema prevail.

The antiquity of sexually-transmitted diseases is unknown, but gonorrhoea is at least as old as the Bible (Wanless 1938; Morris 1946), which means it has been around since at least 1500 BC. According to Morris (1946), references to a disease that was probably gonorrhoea appeared in ancient Chinese writings dating back to 3000 BC. That gonorrhoea was prevalent in North Africa at least 3000 years ago seems firm, however. Since there are no barriers impeding spread of the disease from North Africa to other parts of the continent, it is possible that gonorrhoea has been a cause of low fertility in sub-Saharan Africa for thousands of years.

The source of venereal syphilis has been the subject of scholarly debate for several centuries. Many believe that venereal syphilis was unknown in Europe before Columbus returned from the New World. Others believe that yaws, endemic syphilis, and venereal syphilis are either different manifestations of the same treponema or evolved from a common organism (McFalls and McFalls 1984). Yaws was already widespread in Africa in the fifteenth century, and Portuguese and Spanish slave traders could have brought it to Europe before Columbus (Willcox 1950). If in fact the different diseases are of common origin, then they may be very old. Pre-Columbian skeletal remains with lesions attributed to treponema are known in the New World. This suggests that the disease would have to have been carried across the Bering Strait more than 10 000 years ago for it also to occur in Africa before the journey of Columbus. On the other hand, migration across the Arctic may have continued after the peopling of the New World.

Proponents of the hypothesis that venereal syphilis was imported from the New World have been difficult to challenge. There is no firm evidence that Europeans had treponemal diseases before the return of Columbus. But pre-Columbian diagnoses of other diseases in Europe, especially leprosy, actually may have been caused by treponema (Willcox 1950). Willcox (1950) noted a number of patients who were diagnosed with sexually-transmitted leprosy.

History in Botswana Yaws tends to be found in the moist tropics (Manson-Bahr 1950; Hunter *et al.* 1976), while endemic syphilis is most common in arid regions (Hunter *et al.* 1976). Neither Manson-Bahr (1950) nor Hunter *et al.* (1976) includes Botswana in the places they mention as having yaws or endemic syphilis. Kuczynski (1949) reported cases of syphilis among children in Botswana in the 1930s and 1940s, suggesting non-venereal transmission of the disease there. Guthe and colleagues (1972) reported that non-venereal syphilis was endemic along the eastern edge of Botswana and in south-eastern Namibia along the south-western border of Botswana. One study (Murray *et al.* 1952, Murray 1957, cited in Nurse and Jenkins 1977) found a high prevalence of endemic syphilis among the Kgalagadi of Botswana. Endemic syphilis was also observed among G/wi and G//ana Bushmen (Nurse *et al.* 1973) but apparently not among !Kung. Correspondence from the High Commissioner in Pretoria led Hackett (1953) to conclude that yaws was not endemic in Botswana or South Africa, although it was known to occur among miners.

Of the ethnic groups in which either of these diseases are known to be prevalent, none lives near Herero. The prevalence of both yaws and endemic syphilis have been correlated with environmental factors, such as poor hygiene, which may explain why it is found in some ethnic groups but not others. Today, venereal syphilis is widespread in Botswana, but the antiquity of syphilis and other venereal diseases among Herero is unknown. Both Vedder (1966a) and Irle (1906, cited in Poewe 1985) suggest that the Nama may have introduced venereal syphilis to the Herero tribes in about 1850 during the Herero–Nama hostilities. In 1928, Vedder (1966a, p. 204) noted the popularity of 'witch doctors' who were mostly 'consulted by sufferers of venereal diseases and by childless women'. Steenkamp (1944) published an essay on the causes of low fertility among Herero and concluded that STDs were responsible for their failure to bear children. Gibson (1959) also noted a shortage of children in the population pyramid that he constructed from a survey of Ngamiland Herero. Because of his small sample size, he was reluctant to conclude that the narrow based population pyramid was a result of low fertility.

Government documents cited in Kuczynski (1949) indicate that venereal diseases were clearly widespread in Botswana in 1940. During field-work in Botswana 1967–8, Harpending noted that Herero women frequently complained of pelvic pain while men frequently asked for treatment of symptoms of gonorrhoea. During our field-work in 1987–9, we heard complaints from only a few women, and they had typically already sought treatment for their symptoms from medical clinics. Consequently, it appears that most Herero are seeking treatment for venereal infections before they cause severe damage. Today, PID is included in the *Medical Statistics* report and thousands of cases of gonorrhoea and syphilis are reported (Ministry of Health 1982).

In sum, there is evidence of a long history of both syphilis and gonorrhoea among Herero. Most certainly, other sexually-transmitted genital tract infections that could lead to PID are prevalent as well. STDs have the potential to affect all child-bearing women in a population. They are also responsive to the type of medical treatment that has become increasingly available in north-western Botswana since the 1960s.

Ecology and behaviour

Much of the current work in human reproductive ecology is about the human response to environmental heterogeneity. Synchrony between female reproductive functioning and variability in resource and activity levels would allow females to adjust the output of progeny to some optimal level (Ellison 1990). Differences in the fat stores and nutritional statuses of women may be responsible for variation in levels of fertility, variation in maternal mortality, and variation in the survivorship of offspring (Huss-Ashmore 1980). For example, fat stores in females may function as energy buffers during pregnancy and lactation (Hytten 1980; Crawford 1980; Harpending *et al.* 1990). Women who space births too closely may deplete energy and nutritional stores, adversely affecting fecundity and the survial of young. In theory, mechanisms regulating fertility should evolve to minimize production of offspring with poor survival prospects.

The critical fat hypothesis (Frisch and McArthur 1974; Frisch 1978) suggested that a minimum fat store was necessary for the onset of menarche and for maintaining menstrual cycling. Under this hypothesis, depleted fat stores following parturition and during lactation among women in marginally nourished populations would cause delayed ovulatory cycling and longer birth intervals. Longer birth intervals cause lower fertility since fewer births can occur in the reproductive span. However, this hypothesis has not found much support in the literature (Johnston *et al.* 1975; Huffman *et al.* 1978; Huss-Ashmore 1980; Bongaarts 1982a). Undernutrition probably has very little effect on Herero fertility since they frequently suffer from obesity (O'Keefe *et al.* 1988).

Breast-feeding patterns can also affect the length of birth intervals and, therefore, can contribute to differences in fertility between populations. Frequent and intense suckling may reduce secretion of gonadotropins and inhibit follicular development (McNeilly *et al.* 1988). Previously, researchers thought lactation suppressed reproductive cycling by causing circulation of high levels of prolactin (Konner and Worthman 1980; Stern *et al.* 1986; McNeilly *et al.* 1988). Women who breast-feed their babies frequently and longer post-partum have prolonged birth intervals. This can lead them to have lower fertility than women who breast-feed less. The contraceptive effect of lactation varies but lasts several months. One of the longest delays associated with breast-feeding patterns on cycling has been found among the Gainj of New Guinea, where the median duration of anovulatory lactation was 20 months (Wood *et al.* 1985).

A population-wide reduction in the frequency and intensity of breast-feeding can potentially cause an increase in fertility (Knodel 1977; Bon-

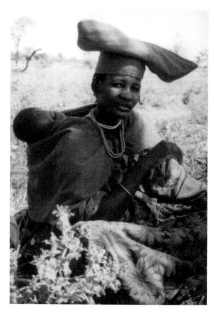

Fig. 6.1. Herero woman carrying infant on back.

gaarts 1981). We do not have careful observations on Herero breast-feeding patterns, but there are no obvious behavioural indications that suggest Herero care for infants differently today than in the past. In our 2 years of field-work, we observed only two Herero women bottle-feeding their infants; one claimed her breasts did not produce enough milk to satisfy her baby and the other was feeding her new-born triplets. Mothers carry their infants tied to their backs throughout the day as shown in Fig. 6.1; they remove the infants and offer them their breasts whenever the infants become restless.

Herero did not express strong beliefs about weaning children, but both young and old women remarked that it was considered correct to wean children only after about 1 year of age. These women said that a child should be weaned if his or her mother becomes pregnant because they consider breast-milk harmful to the nursing child. Even if she has not become pregnant again, many mothers wean their children in their second year of life and give them to relatives to rear (see Chapter 8). We noted that supplementary foods, such as corn porridge and butter, were commonly offered and accepted by infants as young as 3 months of age. While the on-demand style of feeding is consistent with the type thought to maximize the contraceptive effect of breast-feeding, early introduction of supplementary foods lessens the effect. We show in Chapter 7 that most Herero women delay 2 or 3 years before having a subsequent birth.

The !Kung are interesting to contrast with the Herero because they live in the same ecological zone but are ethnically very different. Nancy Howell's (1979) careful demographic study of the !Kung indicated that they spaced their births 4 years apart, and some !Kung were seen breast-feeding 5-year-old children. Because prolonged breast-feeding delays ovulatory cycling, a number of researchers have proposed a variety of adaptational explanations for the wide !Kung birth spacing. A few researchers have hypothesized that !Kung women breast-feed longer due to shortages of suitable bush foods for weaning or because women could carry only one infant on foraging trips (Bleek 1928; Lee 1979). Others have suggested that !Kung who space their births widely have increased reproductive success because they have reduced mortality among their young (Blurton Jones and Sibly 1978; Blurton Jones 1986). Pennington and Harpending (1988), however, found no association between the fertility of !Kung women and the survivorship of their offspring.

Prolonged lactation undoubtedly contributes to wide birth spacing among !Kung. The causal direction of the relationship between lactation and long birth intervals, however, is obscured in longer intervals. For example, !Kung women wean their children once they recognize that they are pregnant again (Howell 1979; Konner and Worthman 1980). Thus, women with low fecundability wean their children at older ages so that prolonged breast-feeding may be an effect rather than a cause of low fertility. Harpending and Draper (1990) have argued that the !Kung, like their Herero neigbours, were afflicted with pathological infertility. In Chapter 9, we contrast !Kung and Herero demographic rates to examine this issue more thoroughly.

Maternal depletion may also constrain female fertility. For example, women who space their births too closely may become nutritionally depleted because they are unable to recover maternal resources between pregnancies (Winikoff 1983; Pebley and DaVanzo 1988; Winikoff and Castle 1988). Maternal depletion has the greatest effect on young, high parity women living in marginal environments. The relevance of maternal depletion studies to human evolution is that depletion is thought to lead to lower survivorship of mothers and their offspring. But support for depletion effects in this context is contradictory. Most studies measure nutritional status using anthropometric measures of fat stores in which it is assumed that women with less fat have lower nutritional status. Some studies have found that women with higher parity are thinner than lower parity women of the same age, but others have not. Even studies showing positive results are inconclusive since the same data are subject to an important alternative interpretation (Winikoff and Castle 1988). Infant deaths shorten birth intervals because they remove the contraceptive effect of lactation. Since the maternal depletion idea predicts that the infants of thin women survive less well, there should be heterogeneity in offspring mortality between thinner and fatter women. Thus, women who start reproduction thin may experience more infant deaths leading them to have higher fertility than their age mates who began reproduction with more fat. In other words, thinness may lead to high fertility instead of high fertility leading to thinness. Although Herero experience substantial heterogeneity in the survivorship of their offspring (see Chapter 3), few are undernourished (O'Keefe et al. 1988).

Discussion of causes of low fertility

The direct and indirect estimates of fertility described in the previous chapter indicate that the Herero were afflicted by abnormally low reproductive rates throughout the first half of this century. Women also experienced truncated reproductive spans in that many ceased reproducing at unusually young ages. There appear to be no ecological or behavioural mechanisms of sufficient historical depth that could account for the low fertility rates and the drastic increase that began in 1957–66. The Herero are staunch traditionalists. Since their flight from Namibia in 1904, they have undergone no drastic social change.

In this chapter, we have examined the most serious diseases occurring in Botswana known to impair fertility. We have evaluated the possibility that tuberculosis, malaria, schistosomiasis, and PID caused low Herero fertility earlier in this century. Of the diseases considered, only PID can produce the pattern of fertility consistent with the pattern observed among Herero. Since PID is commonly the outcome of untreated STDs such as gonorrhoea in women, PID has the capacity to affect all child-bearing women in a population. Although the other diseases may be responsible for some loss in fertility, none are likely to produce the population-wide levels of early sterility observed in Herero, and the increase in fertility has not coincided with declines in their prevalences.

In other areas of Africa, PID has been implicated as the major cause of infertility among women seeking medical treatment for infertility (Belsey 1976; Mabey et al. 1985; Cates et al. 1987). Some researchers are reluctant to believe that STDs are responsible for low levels of fertility throughout Africa. They point out that in many regions high frequencies of STDs do not correspond to low fertility rates (Belsey 1976; Caldwell and Caldwell 1983; Doenges and Newman 1989). However, current infection rates are most likely different than they were when the women became sterile years ago. Also, areas reporting high prevalences of STDs tend to be areas where women are being treated for them. STDs do their damage when they are not treated, and their effects on fertility are expected to be greatest where medical treatment is lacking.

Soon after the advent of penicillin in the 1940s and its efficacy against treponema was proven, the World Health Organization staged an extensive anti-yaws campaign in several African countries (Guthe 1962; Guthe *et al.* 1972). In 1950–60 alone, the WHO injected 17 million people in 15 African countries with massive doses of long-acting penicillin. As an indirect consequence of the WHO efforts and other improvements in public health care facilities, the prevalence of STDs declined (Guthe 1962) and fertility in many areas increased (Caldwell and Caldwell 1983). Easy access to antibiotics for treatment of STDs became available to Herero in the early 1960s. Then, mobile medical dispensaries began making regular visits to remote areas of Ngamiland (van Dam and Molosiwa 1987). Since there has been a hospital in Maun since the 1930s (Fako 1984), control of STDs with penicillin may have been under-way sooner in other parts of Ngamiland. There are now permanent health posts staffed with trained nurses in even the most remote areas of Ngamiland.

Accepting the sequelae of STDs as the major cause of low fertility rates among Herero, the fertility increase in 1957–66 reflects a decline in the pace of secondary sterility. In other words, the change in fertility is due to more women having longer reproductive spans rather than still-fertile women becoming more fecund. Especially before the appearance of penicillin-resistant strains of STDs, administration of antibiotics at dispensaries would drastically reduce the incidence of pathological sterility resulting from the sequelae of pelvic infections in women. Consequently, women who became sexually active after about 1960 (those born after about 1945), when treatment became available, would be at lower risk of becoming infertile than women born before then. These women are the first to have access to treatment. Those who became menopausal before 1960 (those born before about 1915) would be the most severely affected since they have been at risk throughout their reproductive spans. Women born after about 1915 would have some advantage since they were able to seek treatment during a portion of their reproductive spans.

We attribute the continued fertility increases among young women after 1960 to increasingly more women seeking treatment for infection and to increases in health services in rural Botswana (Ministry of Health 1982). The higher fertility of the youngest cohort of post-reproductive women is consistent with the suggestion that women reproducing in the 1960s would benefit from the introduction of antibiotics. Few women born before 1921 would benefit from access to the dispensaries introduced in the 1960s. These women had significantly lower CFSs than the two younger cohorts of post-reproductive women. Indirect estimates of the parity of informants' mothers confirm the antiquity of infectious infertility among Herero. Since fertility among the oldest mothers of informants appears to be higher than the fertility of younger mothers, it appears that the cause of sterility became firmly established around the turn of the century.

The history of sub-fertility in Africa

Caldwell and Caldwell (1983) believe that the pathologically low levels of fertility observed throughout sub-Saharan Africa must be relatively recent. They argue that mortality has been so high in Africa that depopulation would be too severe to sustain a long history of pathologically low fertility. They base their position on the assumption of extremely high mortality rates throughout Africa summarized by a life expectancy at birth ($\overset{o}{e}_0$) of only 25 years. The estimates of Herero mortality clearly contradict the generality of this assumption. The Herero $\overset{o}{e}_0$ before 1966 was 51 years (see Chapter 4). Since few government public health programmes had been implemented in western Ngamiland before 1960, there is no reason to believe that mortality in the past was substantially higher. We also know that Bantu speakers in western Africa began colonizing new territories about 3000 years ago (see Chapter 1). The movement of populations into new territories indicates that the African environment is fully capable of supporting rapid population growth.

That Africa was a sparsely populated continent 50 years ago is undisputed. To what extent low population growth is historically due to low fertility vs high mortality, however, is questionable. Given the spread of trade throughout the continent (Phillipson 1985) and the antiquity of gonorrhoea in North Africa, it is not reasonable to assume that gonorrhoea and other STDs did not spread as well. Unfortunately, it is unknown how long low levels of fertility have persisted or what levels of mortality are usual. There are few reliable African demographic data before 1950.

Demographers have assumed that the currently high population growth rates in Africa are the result of declining mortality resulting from post-war improvements in health care. Our estimates of Herero fertility and mortality, however, indicate that improvements in health care have had a much more substantial impact on fertility than mortality. Female $\overset{o}{e}_0$ has increased by less than 25 per cent (Chapter 4). In contrast, fertility has nearly tripled. Holding fertility constant, we show in Chapter 10 that the declines in mortality produce smaller changes in the Herero intrinsic growth rate than the changes in fertility. Throughout Africa, $\overset{o}{e}_0$ in the 1950s was about 40 and is now about 50 (Hill and Hill 1988).

Frank (1983) also examined the impact of sub-fertility on population growth by estimating shortfalls in fertility produced by infertility. Because many women still suffer from involuntary sterility, some researchers predict continued increases in fertility in many parts of Africa (Frank 1983;

Bongaarts *et al.* 1984). Desire for large families remains high in Africa, and childlessness is a heartfelt tragedy (Caldwell and Caldwell 1987). The persistence of high fertility in Africa and among Herero is also interesting because fertility appears to be increasing in the face of declining mortality and improving economic prospects.

Conclusions

In the last chapter, we documented unusually low rates of fertility among Herero. Throughout the first half of this century, many women apparently experienced truncated reproductive careers. Since about 1960, TFRs have increased from 2.65 to 7.02. The CFS of women and the mothers of people we interviewed indicates that fertility was higher in the late nineteenth century than in the first two decades of this century. The increases in fertility in the period 1957–66 coincide with the appearance of rural health posts in north-western Botswana and the dispensing of antibiotics. After considering the effects of various diseases, we believe the sterilizing effects of pelvic infections, such as STDs, caused low fertility in Herero women.

We also examined the importance of ecological and behavioural factors, such as breast-feeding practices and nutrition, on Herero fertility. While these factors undoubtedly account for some of the variation in fertility among Herero women, their importance is overshadowed by the apparent effect of sterilizing disease. Some researchers have argued that nutritional stress has played an important role in the evolution of human reproductive patterns. This study suggests, however, that disease may have a greater impact on female fertility than nutritional status.

Finally, analyses of Herero fertility and mortality suggest that increases in health care may have a more substantial effect on fertility than mortality. Our analyses of Herero vital rates indicate that minor improvements in health care have resulted in a nearly three-fold increase in the birth-rate while survivorship has increased by only a few years. These trends suggest that decreases in sterility rather than increases of survivorship are responsible for transforming the African continent into one the fastest growing regions in the world.

7

Life history and marriage

Introduction

Demographers and anthropologists typically consider marriage the normal context for child-bearing in human societies. Common approaches to dealing with non-marital reproduction are to ignore it because it is rare or to treat it as an abnormality that requires an explanation. Because there are no universal biological or social constraints limiting reproduction to marital unions, we are hesitant to adopt this view. Instead, we suggest that marriage and reproduction are understood by viewing them as concurrent rather than equivalent states of the life course such that one state is affected by the other but is not dependent upon it. Since a reproductive advantage conferred by marriage can vary among individuals and across ecological and social environments, rather than trying to understand why women do not marry, we might just as well ask why they marry at all.

Apart from the purely social side of human mating, reproductive behaviour is the product of evolution. When to reproduce and how fast are important variables in the life history of all species. In the case of humans, early and rapid reproduction may confer a cost in terms of the survival of mothers and their young and in terms of longevity. The risk of mortality to both mothers and new-borns is J-shaped, being highest at the youngest and oldest ages of mothers (Heady and Daly 1955; Yerushalmy et al. 1956; Nortman 1974). Closely spaced births have been correlated with higher offspring mortality (Yerushalmy et al. 1956; Wray 1971; Federick and Adelstein 1973; Wolfers and Scrimshaw 1975; Hobcraft et al. 1983; Palloni and Tienda 1986; Pebley and Stupp 1987), and high parity especially at young ages has been correlated with shorter female life-spans beyond the reproductive years (Begon and Mortimer 1986). For these reasons, the focus of many public health policies is to reduce teenage pregnancies and parity and to increase the spacing of births to promote the health of women and their children. From an evolutionary perspective, however, these goals may conflict with the biological propensities of individuals to propagate their genes. For example, despite the excess risk of mortality, individuals who reproduce early and fast may still leave relatively more copies of genes to future generations because of the greater reproductive value of surviving offspring in growing populations (Stearns 1976; Stearns 1977; Horn and Rubenstein 1984). Moreover, individuals who delay child-bearing risk failing to reproduce at all since they may still die of other causes. It is interesting that the higher risks associated with younger and faster repro- duction are not unique to humans (Williams 1966). Moreover, later ages at sexual maturity and longer life-spans are general features of mammals (Williams 1966; Stearns and Crandall 1981), and there is some evidence that early menopause is associated with a reduced life-span (Phillips 1989).

The biological perspective contrasts sharply with the standard approach taken by social scientists. Many studies of the biology of fertility distin- guish among women in different marital states to account for women in poor risk categories who might cause the 'true' pattern of natural fertil- ity to look wrong. For example, fertility studies often exclude unmarried women because variation in levels of fertility has been correlated with mar- ital status (Leridon 1977; Bongaarts and Potter 1983). Unmarried women may have lower fertility because they are rarely exposed to coitus, but the causal connection between marital state and fertility is sometimes ambigu- ous. An examination of other factors affecting the life courses of individ- uals might lead us to create different and possibly more useful categories to predict female fertility in other contexts. In many parts of sub-Saharan Africa, marital status is a weak predictor of fertility as many children are born to unmarried women (Fig. 7.1. Apparently, the costs and benefits of reproducing in various marital states are not universal.

The purpose of this chapter is to understand the role of marriage in Herero reproduction. Most Herero women begin producing offspring before marriage such that nearly 40 per cent of all children are born to unmarried women. In this context, we describe several strategies available to Herero men and women for producing and supporting progeny. Because marriages are unstable, many Herero move in and out of the various marital states several times in their lifetimes, and few know the years of their marriages and divorces. We estimate the years of these events from the birth years of offspring and assumptions about their timing in the life cycle. We quantify the effects of alternative life courses on the reproductive performance of Herero women using logistic regression and multivariate life table methods that measure differences in fertility between married and unmarried women of various ages and parity. Our results show that a woman's fertility is affected by her marital status but in an unexpected way. Married and unmarried women in stable marital states have birth intervals of the same length. However, Herero women who change marital states following a birth have poorer prospects of giving birth again than the women who either stay married or unmarried. In addition, the length of women's birth intervals do not appear to affect their chances of becoming married or unmarried. This means that women with high fertility are not more likely to be married than women with low fertility and that low female fertility does not cause

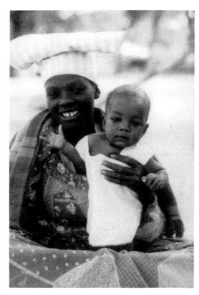

Fig. 7.1. Young unmarried woman with infant.

couples to separate.

The context of Herero reproduction

Marriage

Like many other sub-Saharan groups, high rates of non-marital fertility characterize the Herero. Thirty-eight per cent of all Herero progeny are produced outside marriage. Although most women marry at some point in their reproductive spans, it is not unusual for them to bear a child or two before marriage. Should they become divorced or widowed, remarriage is not prerequisite for continued child-bearing. Men acquire children through marriage, as they are guaranteed rights in the children born to their wife or wives while they are married to them, whether or not they are their genitors. In addition, they may also purchase (with cattle) patrilineal rights in the children of their unmarried girlfriends. Herero may also acquire foster children from their relatives, or, alternatively, may find relatives to rear their children for them. Thus, there are clear alternatives to marriage for both Herero men and women for biological and social reproduction.

Out-of-wedlock child-bearing does not seem to affect a woman's chances of marrying. In fact, we met a number of women carrying children fathered by other men at the time of their marriages, although it is more common for women to have children with men they later marry. However, it is

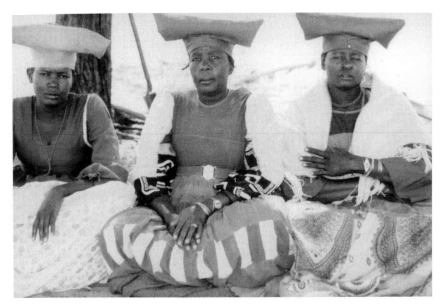

Fig. 7.2. Three Herero co-wives.

our impression that children are not the primary reason marriages between couples are arranged. The majority of first births (55 per cent) are to unmarried women, indicating that many women do not marry until several years after they are sexually mature. Herero males marrying for the first time tend to be several years older than their wife. Men commonly marry more than one wife in their lifetime (see Fig. 7.2), especially if they become divorced or widowed, though a few do not marry at all. The combined effect of a differential age at marriage and the practice of ageing men taking additional wives of reproductive age means that women are often much younger than their husbands (see Fig. 7.3). Women thus have a good chance of becoming widowed during their reproductive years.

Herero marriage is unstable. Many Herero told us that marriages are arranged by elders and that individual partner preference is not an overriding consideration. The ideal mate for a Herero is a cross-cousin. According to Gibson (1959) and Schapera (1945), Herero marriage is exogamous with respect to both matrilineage and patrilineage. Our research and Schapera's, however, indicate that the exogamy rule is not strictly followed (see Chapter 1). Ideally a man marries the daughter of his father's sister, though any cross-cousin will do, especially of his father's matrilineage. Bride-wealth is about three cattle. Herero bride-wealth was traditionally a standard amount, being either one ox, one heifer and four sheep, or one ox and

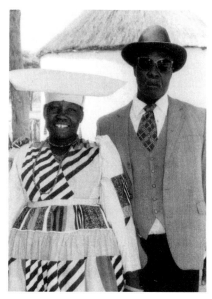

Fig. 7.3. Married Herero couple.

two cows (Gibson 1959). The ox is eaten at the marriage feast. However, we heard of bride-wealths consisting of a combination of an ox, cows, calves, goats, sheep and other livestock and cash. In any case, there is not a substantial variation in the value of bride-wealth, especially considering the large herds owned by some Herero and the fact that bride-wealth in other pastoral groups is frequently about ten to twenty cattle (Gibson 1962). In addition, payment is often waived for marriages between close relatives. Men may also purchase women on credit, but the patrilineage of the woman's father may claim children born during the marriage if the bride-wealth is not paid.

Gibson (1959) says that bride-wealth (*otjitunja*) is for children, but the amount is the same for wives of all ages, including those who are post-reproductive. Gibson also wrote that marriages are legitimized not by the payment of bride-wealth but by the occurrence of the *onjova* ceremony, which involves the ritual slaughter of a sheep at the bridegroom's homestead. Interestingly, a standard child-price is three cattle, perhaps substantially more than bride-wealth since none of it is consumed at the marriage ceremony and it gives men no rights in women.

Herero practise wife inheritance, the levirate, and the sororate (Gibson 1959). With the levirate, the widow may take one of the deceased husband's classificatory brothers as her husband, and the children she subsequently has are in the deceased husband's name. With wife inheritance, the result-

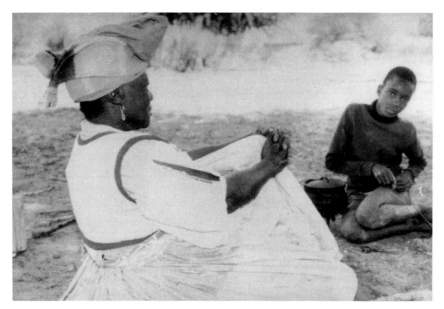

Fig. 7.4.   A Herero wife with the young girl she married to her husband.

ing children belong to the new husband. We do not know to what extent in practice Herero distinguish between these as in both cases the new husband is a member of the deceased's patrilineage. With the sororate, a sister of a wife replaces the wife. If a wife is sterile, she may go to her people and get a new wife for her husband to breed in her place (see Fig. 7.4). The sororate may also occur if a wife dies. In both cases the replacement wife acquires the status of the original wife. This custom provides a way for a sterile wife of a rich man to divert cattle of her husband to her own family.

We do not know what causes Herero marriages to break down. We heard of some marriages in which the couples divorced because one of the partner's families disliked the spouse. The salient characteristics reported by Herero in good matches, in addition to genealogical ties, are hard work and obedience in a wife and ability to provide in a husband. Mutual respect and affection are also important. Women are valued helpers and provide children for a homestead. Men who do not value their women and treat them poorly will cause their wives to leave and suffer for it.

Social and biological reproduction

A stark Darwinian view of human behaviour is that individuals are designed to maximize their own fitness as well as that of their kin. But when there are heritable resources, the ultimate or long-term fitness of an individual

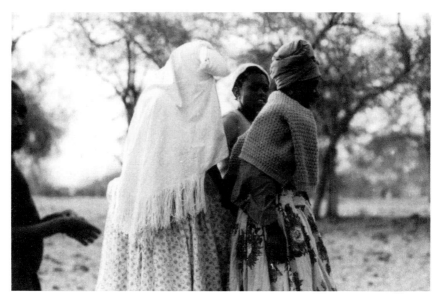

Fig. 7.5. New Herero bride being received at her husband's homestead.

may bear little relationship to a single generation fitness. Someone who has many offspring but cannot provide resources for these offspring may have few or no grandchildren (Rogers 1990; Harpending and Rogers 1990). Further, it seems that cultural transmission can generate seemingly maladaptive individual behaviours, so that individuals may be more concerned with social rather than biological reproduction.

Because the Herero have both matrilineages and patrilineages, individuals belonging to the same patrilineage may belong to different matrilineages and have opposing reproductive and economic interests. While the patrilineages are local and weak, matrilineal relationships are widespread, salient, and important in brokering social relationships. A Herero woman adopts the patrilineal customs of her husband when she moves into his homestead at marriage (see Fig. 7.5) while they both retain the matrilineages they acquired at birth (see Chapter 1). Since Herero marriage is ideally exogamous with respect to matrilineages, men must negotiate culturally sanctioned obligations to a wife's matrikin while maintaining connections to his own lineage groups. Since cattle are ideally managed by the patrilineal homesteads, a man must manage the competing economic interests of the matrilineages of his homestead.

Our own theoretical orientation is that human culture is a system of beliefs that are constrained by the evolved abilities and propensities of humans but that they are not necessarily or even usually (biologically)

adaptive for individuals. As in other societies, there are culturally defined goals that may penalize fitness. A fruitful approach to understanding
constraints on culture might be to study culture with explicit attention
to the tension between cultural and biological goals, and there appear to
be distinct differences between the sexes. For example, in interviews with
Herero about reproductive histories, women name their biological children
while men name their dependents. In the context of parental care and investment, women speak of the importance of 'blood' while men speak of
responsibilities to their dependents and to their patrilineage.

The male focus is on the patrilineal homestead. Large homesteads seem
to be a source of pride as they indicate the extent of a lineage's followers
as well as its wealth. Men place so much value on children that they view
children that their wives have with other men during their marriages as
bonuses, not embarrassments. 'The children are still mine', they say.

A man's focus on social reproduction does not come about until after
marriage, and most men do not marry until they are into their 30s. Meanwhile, they may concentrate on biological reproduction by having children
with girlfriends, and they may purchase patrilineal rights in these children
with cattle. These children become legal children of the father and belong to his lineage, although their status is said to be junior to all marital
children, even those not yet born. If the children have not already been fostered out, men may bring their purchased children back to their homestead
and have their mothers or wives rear them.

The child-price (*okatjivereko*, Gibson 1956) is two or three cattle and
gives a man patrilineal rights in all the children that he has with a woman
in the same way that the payment of bride-wealth gives a man rights in the
children his wife has. The amount of child-price was apparently less until
the Tswana courts ruled that the Herero must pay an amount equal to
bride-wealth (Gibson 1956). The final bill for non-marital children can be
substantially greater than bride-wealth, however, as men may be charged a
seduction fee of ten or twenty cattle if they impregnate very young girls. A
man may pay the seduction fee without purchasing rights in his children.

Men are not guaranteed rights in their non-marital children. Some
complained that they were not permitted the privilege of purchasing their
children and that they were even denied the news of them. This is not
to say that all men desire their non-marital children, and some women
complained bitterly that the father of their children refused responsibility
for them. Unpurchased non-marital children belong to the patrilineage of
their mother's father so that brokerage of these children may be important
for establishing alliances among lineage groups. The putative fathers of
roughly half of all non-marital children of both sexes eventually claimed
their children. Some children were already adults or deceased by the time
their fathers claimed them, but 46 per cent of all non-marital children

in our database who were at least 10 years old were claimed. Thus, the proportion of children who are not supported by their putative biological father is small.

From a woman's point of view, having non-marital children may be an attractive option, especially if she has them with several different men from whom she can collect child-price. However, there is no guarantee that a boyfriend will want to claim his children or that her elders will allow it. In addition, a single woman who fails to give birth will have no means of support apart from her own resources. While a woman may receive gifts from lovers to help, without official ties she may not always call upon them in times of need, especially if they already have wives to support. Even if a lover claims his children, the children are junior to children he has through marriage and may receive truncated inheritances. In sum, staying single can be economically risky for a woman. Through marriage, however, a woman may acquire resources such as cattle from her husband. A wife may also rely on the support network of her husband in addition to her own. On the other hand, Herero women are capable of owning large herds of cattle. Although some have argued that a woman's cattle really belong to her male relatives, she in fact has a say in the management of her cattle and receives the proceeds when they are sold. Thus, there may be fewer advantages to marriage for women from rich families.

Clearly, there are a number of factors that can influence the reproductive choices of Herero men and women. An obvious but hard to answer question is whether there is any reproductive advantage to any particular strategy. We attempt to answer this question by comparing the fertility of married and unmarried women at various points in their reproductive span. Although we can never know how a woman would have fared had she chosen a different life course, we hope to show whether marital status is correlated with child-bearing among Herero women. We ignore males because they were not reliable informants about their biological reproduction.

Does marriage increase fertility?

There are different ways of understanding the relationship between marriage and fertility. One way is to describe it numerically as demographers do, another is to try to understand its social context (Sween and Clignet 1978; Draper 1989). For example, demographers focus much of their research on measuring correlates of fertility differentials that may or may not imply a causal relationship, or on understanding population dynamics, such as age–sex structure, that make attributes such as polygyny possible (Chojnacka 1980; Goldman and Pebley 1989). The first part of this chapter took the latter perspective and investigated the social context of Herero marriage by considering the competing and often conflicting reproductive goals among lineage groups and between the sexes. Our conclusion is that there is more than one acceptable context in which Herero reproduction can occur and that women may choose either or both of them. Our task here is to measure how these alternative life courses are related to the fertility of Herero women.

An interest in the relationship between marriage systems and fertility differentials has a long history in the social sciences. A number of studies have found that co-wives have different fertility (Dorjahn 1958; Shaikh *et al.* 1987; Smith and Kunz 1976; Ukaegbu 1977; Pebley and Mbugua 1989; Sween and Clignet 1978). Some researchers have speculated that polygynously married women have lower fertility because a husband must divide his time among his wives (Musham 1956). Although coital frequencies do seem to affect a woman's chances of conceiving, the importance of this on the population level has not been established (Wood and Weinstein 1988). Other researchers have observed that post-partum sexual taboos, which increase the length of birth intervals, are more strictly observed in polygynous unions, thereby causing these women to have lower completed fertility (Dorjahn 1958; Dorjahn 1959). Many studies can be criticized on methodological grounds. Some do not account for the older age of women entering polygynous marriages or even the age differences between senior and junior wives, and a number of studies have been able to attribute most of the variation in fertility levels related to polygyny to such factors (Ahmed 1986; Bean and Mineau 1986; Borgerhoff Mulder 1989; Pebley and Mbugua 1989).[1] In parts of sub-Saharan Africa having high levels of infertility, birth cohorts experiencing various degrees of infertility would confound differences in fertility among co-wives.

The abundance of literature attempting to link polygyny with variations in fertility levels exemplifies the widespread notion that marriage is the outstanding determinant of fertility. In many and possibly most non-contracepting populations, married women have higher fertility than unmarried women. For this reason, demographers often summarize reproduction using total marital fertility rates computed from age-specific marital fertility rates (Knodel 1983), and population measures of proportions of women married at various ages are used to project fertility levels. However, there are numerous exceptions, particularly in sub-Saharan Africa. With about 40 per cent of all births occurring to unmarried Herero women, we clearly would be overlooking something important about reproduction if we discounted unmarried women. The Herero are not at all unique. African censuses typically distinguish between the fertility of married and ever married women. While these categories do capture distinctive

---

[1] An analysis similar to Ahmed's with apparently the same data set was published a year later by Aborampah (1987). Adepoju (1978) also arrived at similar conclusions regarding a predominantly Yoruban group of women.

population features, they reveal very little about the processes generating them. It is possible that a better understanding of the underlying processes may lead us to construct different, more informative categories when they are needed. For example, the exploratory analysis we conduct below suggests that a more informative classification might be 'ever unmarried' and 'other'.

Unfortunately, we lack an appropriate method for partitioning marital and non-marital fertility. Divorce and widowhood are common among Herero so that many women move in and out of the married state several times during their reproductive spans, and only a few Herero were able to report their years of marriage and divorce. Ideally, we would also like to know how polygyny fits in, but most women did not know much about other women who had divorced their husbands or who were deceased.

Many Herero cannot read or write, but most are able to provide the years of vital events, such as the years of birth of themselves, their children, their spouses, and their parents and the years of death of family members using the Herero year names described in Chapter 2. Herero typically name years after some event occurring in that year, which begins with the rains. These year names have been aligned with Gregorian years and were used to date many of the vital events in our analyses. Although it might be possible to obtain the years of marriages and divorces using the year names, most people simply do not consider these events important and do not bother to remember them. However, women are able to report whether each birth occurred within marriage or not. For women who reproduce throughout their reproductive spans, we can estimate the years of marriages and marital dissolutions from the birth years of their children. For example, a woman having a marital birth subsequent to a non-marital birth became married at some point between these births, and women having a non-marital birth subsequent to a marital birth became divorced or widowed during the interval.

However, this method is less suitable for estimating the years of marital events for women with long birth intervals or for women whose first births occurred relatively late in reproduction. For example, the year of marriage of a woman who had her first birth at age 30, and who was known to be married at the time of the birth but for an unknown period, cannot be reasonably estimated. Similarly, a divorced woman who had only one birth while she was young and married and never had another usually was not able to tell us the year her divorce occurred. In many cases we also had difficulty distinguishing the sequence of divorce, widowhood, and menopause. Many old women reported to us that they were divorced and that the husband was now dead but in an unknown year. Death, especially of spouses, is a sensitive subject, and we were reluctant to and often discouraged from probing this issue in more detail. Many women simply did not remember whether they were post-reproductive by the time they were divorced. Consequently, it is difficult to determine which years of a woman's reproductive span were spent never married, married, divorced, or widowed. Since it is not uncommon for a Herero woman to return to her kin when she is post-reproductive, either because she has become sterile pathologically or naturally, marital dissolution and infertility may not be independent.

We deal with these limitations by ignoring the first birth interval (time to the first birth) and by distinguishing between two types of marital states only, married and unmarried. Ignoring the first birth interval is probably inconsequential. Many Herero women do not marry until several years after puberty, and the majority (55 per cent) of first births are to unmarried women. Because getting married and having a birth for the first time are competing events, unmarried women having their first birth tend to be younger than women who do not have a first birth until they are married. However, if the reproductive opportunities of a woman are affected by her marital status, we may overlook something interesting by collapsing three types of unmarried states into one.

Hazard models

A way to measure fertility differentials is to estimate the probability that a woman has a birth as a function of her marital status. We handle birth intervals during which women experience changes in marital states by treating marital status as a time-varying covariate. Our first step is to select a model with which to estimate the hazard λ_t that a woman has a birth in the tth year since her previous birth. Ideally, we would choose a hazard function that describes the 'true' failure rate, but since we do not know what this is, we settle for an approximation. In practice, the choice of a hazard function has little effect on the estimate of the covariates (Allison 1984). This appears to be true for our problem as well.

The natural shape of the hazard of having a second or higher ordered birth is non-monotonic. After giving birth, women experience 1–3 three months of post-partum amenorrhoea. Return of menses and ovulation is further delayed in breast-feeding women. Herero women breast-feed their infants on demand for at least a year so that most women are infecund for several months after a live birth. Once a mother resumes cycling, she is likely to experience a waiting time until she reconceives even if she experiences intercourse regularly. Thus, even in the absence of pregnancy wastage, the hazard of having a next birth is low immediately following a birth, after which it increases. The most fecund or exposed women give birth again soonest so that as time goes on the hazard declines to zero, when only women who have become sterile are still at risk of giving birth. The simplest hazard model of this form is a quadratic that depends on time

t and t^2.

In addition to time and marital status, there are numerous factors that predict the length of birth intervals. Our purpose is not to identify all of them, but rather to make sure that the power of another characteristic of women that effects the length of birth intervals is not captured in the variable of marital status. We choose to incorporate age at previous birth and birth year of previous child into our model since these variables have substantial effects on the length of birth intervals and might obscure the effect of marital status. Later, in a separate analysis, we incorporate birth rank of previous child as a variable. Because a woman's age and parity are highly correlated, we ignore parity in the following analysis.

Deciding when women are married or not

We treat marital status as a time varying covariate, which means that at each year t of the birth interval, marital status can take on different values. There is nothing mysterious about incorporating time varying covariates in hazard models except, it is the case, however, that easy-to-use statistical packages that can estimate these models have only become available recently.

Since we did not know the years of marital events, we used the marital state at the beginning and ending of intervals as guides. A woman's initial marital state was determined by the type of her previous birth. Obviously, a woman who remains married or unmarried throughout a birth interval of length x spends each year $t, t = 1, \ldots, x$, married or unmarried. We will refer to these types of birth intervals as *continuous* and to intervals during which a woman changes her marital status as *mixed*. We considered women in leviratic marriages to be continuously married since in actuality they never enter an unmarried state. A woman who remained in her husband's homestead after his death but who did not become the wife of a brother of the deceased husband was considered to have become unmarried, even if she continued to give birth in her husband's name.

For women with mixed birth intervals longer than one year, we assumed that the change in marital state occurred exactly at the midpoint of the interval.[2] Therefore, a woman who was married at the beginning of the interval but who was unmarried when she had her next birth or when she was censored was assumed to have spent the first half of the interval married and the last half unmarried. Women who were unmarried but became married during the interval were assumed to have spent the first half of the interval unmarried and the last half married. We assumed the same about women who had censored birth intervals of 1 year. However, we assumed that women who had closed birth intervals of 1 year, spent

---

[2]This assumption will be relaxed later.

the entire year in their final marital state. We assumed that births and deaths always took place at the end of a year, in that order, so that any woman known to be alive in a year was considered to be at risk the entire year. Since births occur at the end of a year, information about the birth intervals of a woman first enters the analysis the year following her first live birth.

There are several problems with these assumptions. First, they imply that women never become married or unmarried in the last half of the longest birth interval. Our longest mixed birth interval is 31 years. Since we assumed that the change in state occurred after 15.5 years, we have assumed that changes in marital state do not occur after women have stayed single or married for 15.5 years of the interval. This is not a realistic model. It is also possible that women who are infertile may be more likely to get divorced. If this were true for the Herero, divorces would be more likely to occur at the end rather than at the middle of an interval. This would also be true if a woman became unmarried due to widowhood since mortality would increase as the husband aged during the interval. Even if a woman's chances of changing marital state were constant, the probability that she experienced a change in martial state by a certain point in her birth interval increases with the length of the interval simply because she has been at risk longer.

There is also the idea that the most fecund women, because of their greater reproductive value, may be preferred marriage partners. Unmarried women with short birth intervals would be more likely to marry during the interval. Demographers often struggle to estimate fecundity from first birth intervals since too many of them are shorter than normal gestation times, suggesting that fertility causes marriage. There is also the idea that women of 'proven fertility' are more desirable wives, so on these grounds we might expect that fertile women are preferentially selected as wives. We might be better off modelling changes from the unmarried to the married state as a function of short birth intervals. On the other hand, we saw from the parity progression ratios in Chapter 5 that, at least among older women, nulliparous women were more likely to be fertile than women who have given birth. Coale (1971) also found that, once a woman reaches marriageable age, her chances of marrying decrease as she ages. This means that changes from the unmarried to the married state would occur at the beginning of intervals. Also, we suggested above that marriage is a less desirable life course for rich Herero women. If there are social class differences in fecundity, we might see the least fertile women choosing marriage. For now, however, we retain our assumptions and consider the possibility of bias later.

Maternal age

Age is one of the most significant factors affecting a woman's fecundity, although the biological basis of this is not fully understood. It is easy to see from looking at the age-specific fertility rates in Chapter 5 that fertility is low early in the reproductive span and gradually increases until it peaks in the mid-20s. It then gradually declines until reaching zero at menopause. Although we combined the experiences of married and unmarried women in our estimates of Herero fertility, the pattern is the same in natural fertility populations when attention is restricted to marital fertility. Fertility is probably low early in the reproductive span because of variability in the age of sexual maturity in girls. Girls undergo a period of 'adolescent sterility' during which they experience irregular cycling that may last several years. This may cause them to have lower fertility than fully mature females. Much of the decline in fertility at older ages may be due to increases in pregnancy wastage, resulting in an increase in the time between live births. Women may also become less fecund as they age, especially if there is a relationship between health and fecundability as there was among Herero women earlier in this century. As women approach menopause, they begin again experiencing irregular cycling until they cease to ovulate completely. In sum, once women become reproductively mature, their chances of giving birth decline as they age.

Concurrent with the decline in reproductive potential, the proportion of births to married Herero women increases with age. For example, 55 per cent of first births are to unmarried women while altogether only 38 per cent of births are to unmarried women. The decline in the proportions may be due either to unmarried women having fewer births or to more women becoming married (or both) as they age. If married women have higher fertility than unmarried women but tend to be older, we might be unable to detect differences in fertility between married and unmarried women if we do not include age as a variable.

The variable *age* refers to a woman's age at the time of her previous birth. We scored age as an ordinal variable with six age classes, ≤ 19, 20–4, 25–9, 30–4, 35–9 and ≥ 40.

Previous child's birth year

In Chapter 5, we described a dramatic increase in fertility among Herero women in the last few decades. Because the fertility transition affects the length of birth intervals, we included a variable to control for the expected differences in risk to women reproducing in different time periods. Some Herero say that marriage practices are weaker than they have been in the past. This claim implies that the high rates of non-marital fertility are a result of fewer women marrying and more women having children outside marriage. At the same time, we have documented an increase in fertility. Since there is a possibility that some of the apparent increases are due to changes in reproductive behaviour, we might confuse this with differences in fertility between married and unmarried women. For example, suppose that married and unmarried women have exactly the same fertility and that there are two periods in which we are measuring fertility, an early and a recent period. Suppose that in the early period, women had an average of two births, while in the recent period they had an average of four. Further suppose that 10 per cent in the early period were unmarried but that in the recent period 50 per cent of women were unmarried. If we collapse over period, our estimate of the number of births per unmarried woman is 3.67 compared to 2.71 for married women.

We used the birth year of the previous birth to control for the effects of time. We scored it as an ordinal variable with six categories, births before 1941, births in 1941–50, 1951–60, 1961–70, 1971–80, and births after 1980. We chose these year intervals to apportion the number of births as evenly as possible into each category.

Estimating the model

There are different ways of estimating the hazard of giving birth; we chose logistic regression. We let λ'_t represent the logistic transformation of the hazard λ_t so that

$$\lambda'_t = \ln \frac{\lambda_t}{1 - \lambda_t}, \qquad t = 1, 2, \ldots, N.$$

The logistic regression model is then

$$\lambda'_t = x_t \alpha, \qquad t = 1, 2, \ldots, N$$

where x_t is a 1×5 vector of covariates (a constant, t, t^2, age, previous child's birth year), and α is a 5×1 vector of its unknown parameters. A property of logistic regression is that as λ'_t varies between $-\infty$ and ∞, λ_t varies between 0 and 1 only, the actual range of probabilites. The coefficients describe how the log-odds change as each covariate changes by one unit(Allison 1984). Although the logistic regression estimates λ'_t rather than λ_t, we can estimate the hazard through substitution. For example,

$$\lambda_t = \frac{1}{1 + \exp(-\alpha x_t)}.$$

We estimated the parameter values of the logit model using maximum likelihood methods. We used an iterative procedure written in GAUSS on a microcomputer. The algorithm chooses values of all the parameters and

Table 7.1. Number of birth intervals contributed by women. We excluded the interval before the first birth in our analysis so
that only women who had at least one live
birth before 1986 contributed data

No. of intervals	No. of women	Total
1	107	107
2	81	162
3	62	186
4	57	228
5	36	180
6	30	180
7	29	203
8	17	136
9	18	162
10	3	30
11	6	66
12	6	72
13	1	13
Total	453	1725

then computes the log-likelihood of the data for each observation year and
its set of covariates using those parameter estimates. The iteration stops
when increases or decreases in the values of any of the parameters no longer
increase the log-likelihood. This is the same algorithm we used to smooth
the mortality rates in Chapter 4 and that Efron (1988) described.

We included in this analysis all birth intervals in which we knew the
marital status of the mother at both the beginning and end of an interval.
This analysis includes information about 1926 live births occurring in 1917
through 1986. Of these, 493 were first births and 72 were twins (16 of which
were first-born). We counted pregnancies resulting in live-born twins only
once. We excluded seventy birth intervals ending in 53 live births because
we were uncertain of a mother's marital status at the beginning and/or
end of an observation. Intervals were censored at the end of 1986 (the year
before the beginning of this study) or when a woman turned 45 or died.
Ninety-five births were followed by intervals of length 0 so that altogether
there were 1725 intervals and 1352 failure events available for analysis. The
number of birth intervals contributed by women is shown in Table 7.1.

Although the excluded birth intervals represent only 4 per cent of the
total number of intervals and failure events, there is some danger that we
introduce bias by omitting these data. However, the excluded intervals constitute the entire birth histories of a small number of women. We obtained

most of these birth histories in our early interviews while still learning to frame our questions to get the information we wanted. For example, a widowed Herero woman who does not remarry names her deceased husband as the father of her children, even though he may have been dead many years when the children are born. While naming a dead man as the father of a child makes perfect sense to a Herero, we do not know whether the woman had a husband during her reproductive years unless we learned when the husband died or asked more questions. In any case, there is no reason to believe that excluded intervals provide different information about births from the data we used. We discuss this issue further when we interpret the results.

Results

The logistic regression described above was used to estimate the effects of a woman's marital status, the year of her previous birth, and her age at the previous birth on her chances of having a next birth. The results are given in Table 7.2. The t-statistics are computed by dividing the parameters by their standard errors. For sufficiently large samples, the t-statistics have a standard normal distribution when the parameter is zero. Using a two-tailed test, values greater than 1.96 have a probability of less than 0.05. All parameter estimates fall well beyond the 0.0001 region of the distribution indicating that it is highly unlikely that their true values are zero. We estimated this model using higher orders of time and significantly improved the fit of the data. For example, removing the square of the duration decreased the log-likelihood to -3191.963. These two models are nested so that twice the difference in their log-likelihoods is approximately χ^2 distributed when the null model is true. The degrees of freedom are equal to the difference in the number of parameters of the two models. The X^2 statistic to test that t^2 is zero is 124.27 on one degree of freedom, $p < 0.000$. Adding terms for higher orders of time resulted in increases of similar magnitude in the log-likelihood. However, these terms had very little impact on the estimates of the coefficients of *previous child's birth year*, *age*, and *marital status*. Since our model is sufficient to tell us what we want to know, we leave it as it is for now. However, if we wanted to smooth the hazard as we did when estimating the hazard of mortality, we would be better off selecting the best model that fit the data.

The parameter estimates indicate that women who gave birth more recently are more likely to give birth again compared to women who reproduced in the past. The parameter estimate says that the logit of a woman's chances of having a next birth increases by 0.245 in each period compared to a woman of the same age and marital status in the preceding period. Similarly, the parameter estimate for the effect of age on fertility indicates that the logit of a woman's chances of having another birth decrease by

Table 7.2. Effects on the length of birth intervals using logistic regression. Changes in marital states in mixed birth intervals were assumed to occur at the midpoint of an interval. We used a dummy variable for marital status in which 0 indicated the married state. The log-likelihood of the model is -3129.829. The probability that any of the parameters is zero is less than 0.0001

Covariate	Estimate	t-Statistic
Unmarried	-0.270	-4.023
Birth year	0.245	10.918
Age	-0.117	-4.927
Constant	-2.051	-14.527
t	0.244	5.726
t^2	-0.035	-8.579

-0.117 as she ages into the next age category, compared to a woman in the preceding younger age class who is of the same marital status and at risk during the same period. In other words, the more recent a woman's previous birth, the more likely she is to give birth again while her chances of giving birth again decline with age. These results were expected. What is surprising is the importance of marital status. We used a dummy variable for marital status (0 is married) to indicate whether a woman was married in each year of her birth interval. The logit of the probability that an unmarried woman gives birth decreases by -0.270 compared to a married woman of the same age at risk during the same period. The effect of this variable is much larger than the effect of age but only slightly larger than effect of previous child's birth year.

How the chances of changing marital state change with time

We are surprised by the importance of marital status and further consider the possibility that the assumptions we used to determine the timing of marital events biased our results. We have already mentioned a number of potential problems with our assumptions. Since the year in which a woman became married or divorced was unknown for most women, we assumed that women who experienced changes in marital states spent an equal number of years in each state. However, it is more natural to assume that changes in marital state are the result of a risk process. By modelling the risk process, we should be able to arrive at better estimates of the timing of events. For example, if the chances that an unmarried woman gets married are either invariant or decreasing through time, most women who become married would do so in the first few years of their birth intervals so that they actually end up spending more than half the length of the birth interval in the married state. If marriages break down because of childlessness such that the risk of becoming unmarried is very low immediately after the previous birth but becomes very high as the length of the interval increases, women who became unmarried may actually spend more than half the interval in the married state. The effect of these factors may have caused us to over-estimate the number of years women spent unmarried in the analysis above. About 65 per cent (164/246) of the mixed birth intervals were of married women becoming unmarried.

We estimated the probabilities of changing marital state from the data by examining the number of women with birth intervals of various lengths who had a change in marital status. We know for each year t the proportion of women with mixed birth intervals who experienced a change by year t. For example, 395 women with birth intervals 2 years long began them unmarried. During the 2 years, 15 of them became unmarried. We can specify a hazard model and then use this kind of information to compute the maximum likelihood estimate of the hazard. If the hazard is a constant p and the length of the birth interval is 2 years, then

$$\frac{p}{p + p(1 - p)}$$

women would be expected to become unmarried in the first year and

$$\frac{p(1 - p)}{p + p(1 - p)}$$

women would be expected to become unmarried in the second year. Under this model, the maximum likelihood estimate of the annual hazard for getting unmarried is 0.019 for the 15 2-year birth intervals so that about half the women would be expected to become unmarried in the first year and half in the second. If we assume that changes in marital state occur at the beginning of a year, then half of the 15 women are expected to spend both years of the birth interval in the unmarried state. The other half spend the first year in the married state and the second year in the unmarried state. By considering the entire data set and assuming a constant hazard (an exponential model), the maximum likelihood estimate of the probability of getting married, given that one is unmarried, is 0.0660 per year, and the probability of getting unmarried, given that one is married, is 0.0194 per year.

Since we suspect that married women are more likely to become unmarried as their birth intervals increase and that unmarried women are more likely to become married if they have short birth intervals, we proceeded to fit the model

$$\lambda_t = e^{\alpha_0 + \alpha_1 t}$$

where λ_t is the probability of getting either married or unmarried in year t and α_0 and α_1 are constants. This hazard, known as the Gompertz, decreases through time from e^{α_0} if α_1 is negative and increases if α_1 is positive. The Gompertz is sometimes used to model human mortality after childhood. If the chance that a married woman gets unmarried increases with the length of her birth interval, then α_1 should be positive. If the chance that an unmarried woman gets married decreases with the length of her birth interval, then α_1 should be negative. However, in both cases our maximum likelihood estimates of α_1 were zero.[3] This reduces the Gompertz to the exponential model that we estimated above. This means that long birth intervals do not increase a woman's chances of becoming divorced or widowed and that short birth intervals do not increase an unmarried woman's chances of becoming married.

We used the probabilities of getting married and unmarried estimated from the exponential model to apportion the years women with mixed birth intervals spent married or unmarried. We assumed that changes in marital status occurred at the very beginning of an interval so that intervals of only 1 year are spent entirely in the second marital state, as they must have been if they end in a birth. We then refit the model in Table 7.2. The results of the new model are given in Table 7.3. It is obvious that going to the extra trouble of apportioning the risk years has made little difference. Although the effect of marital status has been reduced, it is still important.

We added the covariates *previous child's birth year* and *age* because we feared that excluding them would confound the effect of marital status. Excluding birth year results in a smaller parameter estimate for marital status of -0.166 (the t-statistic is -2.514). This indicates that if one ignores birth year of the previous child, the difference in fertility between married and unmarried women appears to be less. If we re-include birth year and exclude age, the effect is similar: the parameter estimate of marital status changes to -0.162 (t-statistic of -2.462). Although excluding these variables would not cause us to reject the hypothesis that marital status does not matter, the effect of marital status would appear to be substantially less.

---

[3]These computations were done using a spreadsheet in Microsoft EXCEL 3.0.

Table 7.3. Effects on the logistic regression when mixed birth intervals are apportioned. The log-likelihood of the model is -3132.993. The probability that any of the parameters is zero is less than 0.0001

Covariate	Estimate	t-Statistic
Unmarried	-0.212	-3.161
Birth year	0.244	10.885
Age	-0.111	-4.735
Constant	-2.087	-14.839
t	0.245	5.764
t^2	-0.035	-8.600

Fertility for different types of birth intervals

Given the large number of births to unmarried women, we are puzzled by the importance of marital status. In an exploratory spirit, we estimated hazardsfor the four different types of birth intervals, continuously married, continuously unmarried, married–unmarried, and unmarried–married. These are plotted in the graph in Fig. 7.6 and are quite revealing. Women who are continuously married or continuously unmarried have nearly identical hazards. However, women who become married or become unmarried during their intervals have much lower hazards, especially married–unmarried women.

Because this investigation is exploratory, we must be cautious in our interpretations. However, the graph does generate some interesting hypotheses. Most intriguing is that unmarried women who have become unmarried since their previous births have the lowest fertility, suggesting that 'stopping rules' may be different for women at this stage in their life course. We showed above that long birth intervals (infertility) do not in themselves lead to the breakdown of marriages, but once a woman becomes unmarried, she may choose to terminate child-bearing if she already has a large number of children. Married women may have little power to refuse their husbands, but they have control over whether they have lovers. This leads us to the hypothesis that women who become unmarried are increasingly less likely to reproduce again as the number of births that they already have increases.

In Chapter 5, we plotted the parity progression ratios of the post-reproductive women in this sample. A parity progression ratio shows the proportion of women who, having had an ith birth have an $i + 1$th birth. The plot of all the progressions produces a concave downwards curve, which

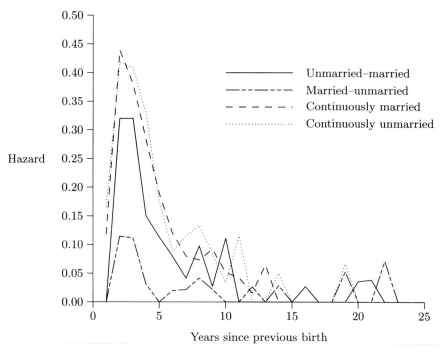

Fig. 7.6. Hazards of giving birth for four types of birth intervals. Women either became married (unmarried–married), became widowed or divorced (married–unmarried), stayed married (continuously married) or stayed widowed or divorced (continuously unmarried) during the birth intervals.

indicates that the probability that a woman gives birth again is not related to the number of births she already has. On these grounds the Herero appear to be a natural fertility population. This does not preclude the possibility that some women at various points in their life cycle may practice alternative strategies that are not detectable in population averages.

Another way of looking at the hazards is by converting them into Kaplan–Meier survivor curves, as we have done in Fig. 7.7. The Kaplan–Meier (product-limit) estimates produce life tables for censored data. If $F(t)$ is the survivor function, n_j is the number at risk at time j, and d_j is the number of births occurring at time j, then the survivor function can be estimated by (Kalbfleisch and Prentice 1980)

$$\hat{F}(t) = \prod_{j|t_j < t} \frac{n_j - d_j}{n_j}.$$

$\hat{F}(t)$ is thus the conditional probability of not giving birth, given that a

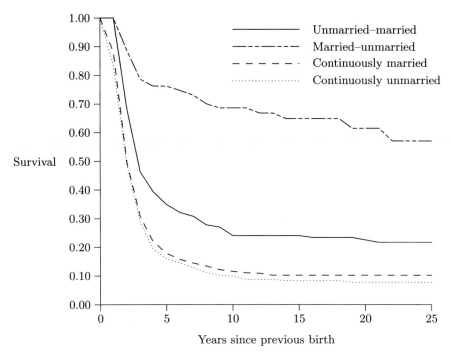

Fig. 7.7. Survivor curves of the hazards of giving birth for four types of birth intervals. Women either became married (unmarried–married), became widowed or divorced (married–unmarried), stayed married (continuously married), or stayed widowed or divorced (continuously unmarried) during the birth intervals.

birth has not already occurred.

We choose to plot these curves because they reflect the cumulative failure probabilities and they asymptote at 1− the parity progression ratios. That is, they show the probability that women in each category have become sterile since their previous birth. The continuous birth intervals level off near 0.1, indicating that the sterility rate is about 10 per cent. The asymptotes of the mixed intervals are much higher, indicating that 20 per cent of women who become married never have a next birth while more than 50 per cent of women who become unmarried never have a next birth. This suggests that a disproportionate number of sterile women have mixed birth intervals. Since the analysis above indicates that there is not a relationship between fertility and the chances that a woman becomes married or unmarried, these results are puzzling, suggesting that a behavioural mechanism is responsible for maintaining low levels of fertility of women once they enter a second marital state. These figures cannot be taken at face value since the effects of other variables, such as age, affect them. However, we show below that the general trend in the data holds even when other factors affecting the lengths of birth intervals are considered.

A proportional hazards model of stopping rules

It is easy to test the hypothesis that women in different marital states follow different 'stopping rules' for having children using a Cox (proportional hazards) model. The Cox regression model assumes a baseline hazard for all individuals but does not specify how the hazard depends on time. Maximum likelihood estimates of covariate parameters are computed under the assumption that the effects of covariates do not depend on time so that the hazards of two individuals varying in one explanatory variable are parallel through time. We used three dummy variables to indicate the four marital states, with the state continuously married being the baseline rate. We included age, previous child's birth year, and previous child's birth rank as covariates as well as three more variables indicating the interaction between marital state and birth rank. Birth ranks range from 1 to 13 (see Table 7.1).

Because some women are either more fecund or better able to carry pregnancies to term, there can be substantial variability in the number of births to same-aged women in natural fertility populations. Throughout the reproductive span, the pace of child-bearing is faster in these extra-fertile women so that, on average, the number of births a woman has at a particular age is a strong predictor of the probability that she will have another birth. However, on an individual level a woman's decision to have a next birth may be affected by her marital state. We model the interaction between marital state and number of previous births by creating three variables in which the birth rank of the previous child is multiplied by each of the marital state indicator variables. We expect to find a negative relationship between cumulative fertility and birth intervals in which women become unmarried and make no prediction about the other types of birth intervals. On the whole, however, cumulative fertility should not negatively affect the probability if the Herero are indeed a natural fertility population. Because only women who have been reproducing for several years can have high parity, cumulative fertility can appear to affect future fertility negatively if the effect of age is not considered as well.

We estimated the proportional hazards model using the SURVIVAL module in the IBM PC version of SYSTAT. The results are given in Table 7.4. The regression estimates do not provide an ounce of support for our hypothesis. In fact, the effect of the interaction between the term for becoming unmarried and birth rank is opposite of the direction expected, although in fact none of the estimates of the interaction terms can be distinguished from zero.

The coefficients for marital status confirm the visual impression of Fig-

Table 7.4. Effects on the length of births intervals using Cox regression. The log-likelihood of the model is −9227.980; † indicates probabilities exceeding the 0.001 region. All the other parameters have probabilities greater than 0.05

Covariate	Estimate	t-Statistic
Birth year[†]	0.145	7.331
Age[†]	−0.130	−4.090
Birth rank	0.033	1.686
Unmarried–unmarried	0.031	0.296
Married–unmarried[†]	−1.108	−3.689
Unmarried–married[†]	−0.763	4.287
Interaction terms:		
unmarried–unmarried × birth rank	−0.013	−0.485
unmarried–married × birth rank	0.039	0.549
married–unmarried × birth rank	0.073	1.244

gure 7.6. The parameter estimate of the effect of being continuously unmarried during a birth interval is not significantly different from zero. Since the model measures deviations from the hazard for continuously married women, this means that the probability of having a next birth is the same for continuously unmarried and continuously married women. In contrast, women with mixed birth intervals have significantly reduced probabilities of having next births. Exponentiating the parameter estimates indicates their relative effect on the baseline hazard. Thus we have that a married woman who becomes unmarried during her birth interval is $e^{-1.108} = 0.330$ times as likely to have a next birth as a continuously married woman, all else being equal. Similarly, the chances that an unmarried woman who becomes married has a next birth is $e^{-0.763} = 0.466$ times that of a continuously married woman. This latter finding also contradicts the idea that fertility causes marriage.

The covariates *previous child's birth year* and *age* agree with the results of the logistic regression models. A woman's chances of having a next birth in a particular period are $e^{0.145} = 1.156$ times what they were in the preceding period. As women age into subsequent age intervals, their risk of having a next birth is only $e^{-0.130} = 0.878$ times what it was in the previous age category. The effect of birth rank is small and statistically not significant. Removing the interaction terms and refitting the model does not change any of the parameter estimates much. The standard error of the birth rank parameter is reduced resulting in a t-statistic of 1.759. However, the standard error is still too large to conclude that the effect is statistically different from zero at the 5 per cent confidence level.

It is interesting that the Cox model produced smaller t-statistics than the logistic regressions. Because the Cox model ignores all information about time in the computation of the parameter estimates, it may produce less efficient estimates (Kalbfleisch and Prentice 1980). However, these may be small (see Efron 1977, and the discussion in Kalbfleisch and Prentice 1980). Although our two models are not directly comparable, some variation between them would be expected due to differences in the parameterization of the marriage effects and because we have assumed that we know how the hazard depends on time. Our experimentation with other parametric models specifying non-monotonic hazards yielded results consistent with both the Cox and logistic models presented here. The biggest differences occurred in the estimates of standard errors. A number of models produced parameter estimates for birth rank that fell well beyond the 5 per cent rejection region. The estimated effects of birth rank, however, remained very small.

Earlier we worried that excluding birth intervals with missing data might bias our results. Although we argued that this is of no consequence, our breakdown of the data into four interval types allows us to state this with more confidence. The relatively low hazard of having a next birth for women who become unmarried is due to a deficit of births that is so large that even if all the births from the missing data fell in that category (which they do not), the hazard would still be substantially lower.

Summary and discussion

Non-marital reproduction tends to be regarded as odd and abnormal. This view may better reflect Western ideals than empirical evidence. Compared to a number of other species, marriage is a weak form of pair bonding. Human parents rarely form enduring bonds founded upon the intense nurturing of offspring observed in many other bisexually reproducing species, most birds and gibbons being the best examples. What we (think we) know about our evolutionary history over the last million years or so also indicates that monogamy is recent and perhaps 'unnatural' (Harcourt *et al.* 1981). A simple Darwinian view suggests that there must be a reproductive advantage to pair bonding for it to evolve and persist. Of course humans are guided by the will of the culture they inherit as well as their genes, but efforts to understand human behaviour as the product of evolution yields insights about human nature that we might otherwise overlook.

In our view, human reproductive behaviour is the outcome of individuals' perceptions of what options are available to them and how they may better or worsen their lot by pursuing any particular strategy or combination of options. The human propensity to observe and learn can either enhance or compromise the biological urge to reproduce that is innate in all animals since some behaviours may enhance long-term fitness at the expense of short term fitness. In any environment there may be some average strategy that reflects the constancy of the ecology, but individuals who vary in their resources and biology may choose alternative life courses.

We discussed the reproductive options available to Herero men and women in the first part of this chapter. Many women produce several offspring outside marriage for their fathers, and the genitors of these children often purchase the patrilineal rights in them. Most women also marry at some point in their reproductive spans during which time they should produce progeny for their husbands' lineages. Similarly, men may obtain children for their patrilineages through unofficial liaisons with girlfriends and through marriage. Non-marital reproduction may be an attractive strategy for women in that they may acquire more cattle for their families than through bride-wealth alone without owing any obligation to husbands. Men must be economically or socially established before they marry, but there are still ways for them to acquire legal children before they are able to marry or as supplements to their lineages. This mode of reproduction may be less costly in that they are not obligated to support the mothers of the children. Non-marital progeny may also be cheaper for men in the sense that they will be junior in status to marital children, even those who are not yet born.

Non-marital reproduction seems to be an attractive reproductive option for both men and women in that both sexes get the children they want at less cost than they might through marriage. However, it is risky. Women who fail to reproduce get nothing and there is no guarantee that the genitors of their children will claim them. Unmarried women must rely on their own resources for support and have a smaller set of relatives to call on in times of need. Moreover, children that are claimed by their genitors are entitled to fewer resources from their fathers than marital offspring. Similarly, men may be denied rights in their non-marital children. In contrast, marriage assures a woman support for herself and her children and may be the surest for a man to acquire children for his lineage.

Since individuals are heterogeneous in the amount of resources they control or have access to, we expect the advantages and disadvantages of either reproductive option (having children married or unmarried) to vary. For example, a woman who is already wealthy will not receive much economic gain through marriage or by allowing her children to be claimed by their genitors, while at the same time her equally rich brother can afford and attract many wives and consorts to produce children for him. At the other end of the economic spectrum women can gain the most by producing progeny for a number of wealthy men and then later marrying. In this way, her family obtains both child-price and bride-wealth. We expect that the poorest males are the least attractive boyfriends and marriage partners. Poor males may have too few resources to afford both girlfriends and wives and probably must choose only one reproductive option if they hope to acquire any children at all.

Unfortunately, we still do not know enough about Herero household economics (Harpending and Pennington 1990) to understand the complexities of Herero mate choice, although this is the subject of proposed future research among them. The Herero are also unusual in that they have a dual-descent lineage system. There can be conflict among closely-related individuals because of tension between the goals of their respective lineages. For example, Herero homesteads are conceptually patrilineal and under the control of the senior male of the lineage. Livestock, especially cattle, are the basis of Herero wealth and tradition. Since men manage the cattle, the unit of production in a Herero household is the patrilineal homestead. In contrast, the consumption units are matrifocal clusters within the homestead. Herero marriage is virilocal and ideally exogamous with respect to matrilineage. As a result brothers who have different mothers belong to different matrilineages but the same patrilineage, and their wives and children will belong to other matrilineages as well. With respect to reproduction, it may be in the interest of the homestead patrilineage to form certain alliances through marriage, but the conflicting goals of their matrilineages may temper any homestead decision.

To gain some insight into the effect of alternative life courses on Herero reproduction, we performed a number of analyses examining the relationship between marital states and fertility. Since about 40 per cent of Herero children are born to unmarried women, we expected that marital status was not correlated with fertility. A survival analysis comparing the probabilities that married and unmarried women give birth again, however, suggests that married women have significantly higher fertility than unmarried women. On the other hand, the fertility differential between married and unmarried women was only slightly greater than the difference in fertility between women reproducing in subsequent time periods (see Tables 7.2 and 7.3).

Few Herero knew the years of their marital events so we restricted our analysis to intervals following the first and higher ordered births and assumed that changes in marital state occurred at the midpoint of intervals. We performed the same analysis using probabilities of the timing of marital events estimated from the data and similar parameter estimates. The lack of differences in the results produced by the two methods illustrates the principal that simple models can produce useful answers. Our estimates of the probabilities that unmarried women get married and that married women get unmarried allow us to reject the hypotheses that fertility is a cause of marriage and that childlessness is a cause of marital dissolutions among Herero. We found that a woman's chances of getting married or unmarried did not depend on the length of her birth interval as would be expected if there were a relationship between fertility and marriageability and marital stability. That there appears to be no obvious relationship between reproductive potential and marriageability supports our notion that reproduction and marriage are not equivalent states. Our claim that infertility does not cause a woman to become unmarried may be confounded because we lumped women who become unmarried due to divorce and widowhood in the same category, but since Herero practise the levirate this may be inconsequential.

An exploratory look at the data suggests that the explanation for low fertility among unmarried Herero women may be unusual. We computed separate hazards for four types of birth intervals. A graph of these hazards (Fig. 7.6) shows that women who stayed married during their birth intervals had virtually the same chance of having a next birth as women who stayed unmarried. However, women who underwent changes in their marital state had substantially lower fertility prospects than women who stayed either married or unmarried. Only about 50 per cent of women who became unmarried (i.e. women who got divorced or widowed) had another birth compared to 90 per cent of women who stayed married or stayed unmarried during their birth intervals. Women who became married have about an 80 per cent chance of having a next birth. These apparent substantial differences in fertility are puzzling since our earlier analysis indicated that changes in marital state were not related to fertility. This suggests that the change in the marital state is the cause rather than the effect of low fertility. Although this finding is provocative, we limit our interpretations to speculation because of the exploratory nature in which our findings were revealed.

None-the-less, the figure does generate a number of interesting hypotheses. We used a proportional hazards model to test one in which we suggested that divorce and widowhood provide ways for women who already have many children to terminate child-bearing, but found no support for it. There is apparently no relationship between the number of births a woman already has and the probability that she will have another one. Women who had higher parity at a given age than others were more likely to have a next birth, but the effect was very small and not significant at the 0.05 level using the proportional hazards model, and there was no correlation between interval type and this effect.

The results suggest other avenues for further research. For example, Gibson (1959) wrote that Herero men are reluctant to marry widowed women because they are afraid that they will die like the other husband. Herero generally attribute the cause of most deaths to sorcery so that corrective measures (i.e. anti-witchcraft) may change this fate. Gibson (1959) also wrote that divorced women are less desirable wives because, according to the Herero, a woman who divorces will divorce again. It would be interesting to see whether these fears in fact resulted in poorer marital and sexual prospects for divorced and widowed women causing them to have lower fertility.

The Herero also say that women who have children before marriage are less desirable wives because they will be thinking about other men during their marriages (Gibson 1959), but both our observations and Gibson's suggest that premarital children do not impede a girl's chances of marriage. Herero men told us they value hard work and obedience most in a wife. A few old men told us that it is proper Herero custom for an old man to have many wives and for these wives to receive male visitors at night because the husband is too old and feeble. It is none-the-less possible that women who reproduce before marriage make less stable marriage partners, especially if they gain economically from the arrangement. These issues could be better addressed if we were able to distinguish between marriages that end by divorce or widowhood.

Perhaps most puzzling is that newly married women have lower fertility. It might be that marriage constitutes a disruption in a woman's life, causing a delay in child-bearing. However, the survivor curves indicate that these women never 'catch-up' to the levels of fertility experienced by women who spend their birth intervals continuously married or unmarried. If it is true that poverty makes marriage a more attractive life course option for women, then the lower fertility might be attributable to poorer health or nutritional status. Fertility differentials in other populations have been attributed to variability in the nutritional status of women (see Chapters 6 and 9). Among the Herero, women who own large herds of cattle have a plentiful food supply, are buffered against drought, and may sell surplus livestock to purchase other goods and services.

Conclusions

Herero fertility is a glaring contradiction to the assumption that reproduction outside marriage is negligible. Although Herero women of reproductive age who are married apparently do have higher fertility than unmarried women, the difference is of the same order of magnitude as the difference in fertility between women reproducing in subsequent time periods.

Our initial analysis indicated that marriage leads to higher fertility, but an exploratory look at the data suggests that the conclusion needs qualifying. Women who undergo a transition in marital state during their birth intervals have the lowest fertility, while women who stay married or unmarried during their birth intervals have identical levels of fertility. In other words, marriage does not increase fertility, rather widowhood and divorce decrease it.

Because of the generally high numbers of children born to women out-side marriage and because of the difficulty in obtaining reliable dates of marital events, African censuses tend to distinguish between women who are either 'ever married' and 'never married'. Our exploratory finding is only suggestive, but indicates that demographers may develop more useful categories by understanding the relationship between marriage and fertil-ity in African social systems. In the case of the Herero, it might be more useful to distinguish between 'ever unmarried' and the rest of reproductive-aged women in the study of fertility. However, we need to substantiate this finding using hypotheses on independent data before drawing any firm con-clusions.

8

Child fosterage and social parenthood

Introduction

Child rearing practices are fundamentally important to our understanding of Herero demography and social ecology because they can be linked to the survival of children, the fertility of women, and the structure and economy of households. Many Herero share their parenting responsibilities with friends and relatives by giving them their children to raise. This custom of child fosterage has a long history in Herero society and is well-known in other parts of Africa (Goody 1982; Frank 1987). Nearly 40 per cent of all Herero are fostered out during childhood.

Child fosterage is relevant to a number of other issues in the social sciences. Exchange of children between households establishes bonds between members of the households and may engender a network of obligations between the biological and foster parents of children. Individuals who take in foster children may receive a source of labour, while individuals who foster out their children may provide new opportunities for their children. In Africa, for example, foster parents living in urban areas can provide schooling for children whose biological parents live in rural areas where there are no schools. Understanding the motivations for child fosterage may be important to understanding household economics.

We became interested in child fosterage because it seemed peculiar to us. Why is a custom so entrenched in African social systems virtually unrecognized in Western nations of the world? Why do the Herero foster out their children while their neigbours, the !Kung Bushmen, do not? We suspect the answers to these questions are related to differences in the advantages of social parenthood in the various societies. To what extent fosterage reflects the demand for foster children vs the demand for foster parents is at the heart of this issue. A number of other studies have stressed the latter perspective, suggesting that mothers foster out their children to increase their fertility (i.e. by weaning their children younger) or to make themselves more attractive to consorts.

In this chapter we examine several prominent themes in the literature about the function of African fosterage in the context of Herero life by looking at the relationship between female fertility and child fosterage rates. We also turn to our own ideas about Herero parenting to understand fosterage. We suggested in previous chapters that sex preferences for children and marriage patterns are closely related to the value of children in Herero society. We observed in Chapter 3 that Herero female infants and children survived two to three times better than males. In Chapter 7 we suggested that women had reproductive roles in both their fathers' and their husbands' households. We relate these observations to sex preferences for foster children and to differences in the number of children that married and unmarried women foster out.

What is child fosterage

Collecting data on child fosterage

The most detailed study of child fosterage that we know of was done by Esther Goody on the Gonja of Ghana. She defined fosterage '... as the institutionalized delegation of the nurturance and/or educational elements of the parental role' (Goody 1982, p. 23). A slightly different definition of fosterage was used by Caroline Bledsoe in her comprehensive studies of child fosterage in Sierra Leone. She defined a foster child as any child living apart from the biological mother (Bledsoe et al. 1988; Bledsoe and Isiugo-Abanihe 1989). Both definitions make arbitrary distinctions, and the usefulness of either depends on the particulars of a population and the question at hand. Demographers can use definitions like Bledsoe's to garner data on fosterage from national survey data that lack ethnographic details but include information about residence of children and their mothers (Frank 1987; Page 1988). This definition, however, ignores the parental role of fathers.

We obtained information on fosterage of 1902 individuals in two ways. First, we asked 519 Herero men and women if they were ever raised by someone other than their biological parents (self-ascertained). Second, we asked the people we interviewed if each of their children had ever been given to someone else to be raised (1539 individuals parent-ascertained). One-hundred and fifty-six of the individuals we interviewed were also ascertained through a parent. Herero said they were 'raised' if their primary caretakers were not their biological parents. We classified all individuals who reported that they or their children were ever 'raised' as fostered. The Herero's criteria for being 'raised' seem to correspond to Goody's definition of fosterage.

We noted occasional discrepancies between self- and parent-ascertained reports, but we cannot assess their importance since we frequently interviewed parents and offspring in each other's presence. For example, a daughter present during the interview of her mother often answered the questions about herself. If the daughter subsequently gave a reproductive history, we would record her as both parent- and self-ascertained. When a discrepancy arose and we could not find all the individuals involved to resolve the discrepancy, we used the self-ascertained response.

When children are fostered out

We classified many children being raised in the same homestead as their biological parents as fostered, because the children would continue to live with the foster parents should either party move out of the homestead and because the children were often fostered out to separate households within the homestead. At divorce, women leave children to whom they gave birth in their husband's homestead but may take with them children that have been fostered to them. Similarly, an unmarried woman who has fostered out a child to a member of her homestead will leave her child with the foster parent when she marries out of the homestead. Most homesteads, which are schematically patrilineal, consist of distinct matrilineal clusters (see Chapter 1). Each matrilineal unit is centred around a mother and the children she raises and in many respects is an economically distinct unit within the larger homestead. Most children fostered within a homestead eat from a different pot than their biological parents and in this sense live in separate households.

Children living in homesteads other than their biological parents' were not classified as fostered unless their biological parents had transferred their care to another adult. Because of their isolation in rural Botswana, Herero children are often separated from their biological parents for long periods. Children from rural areas live in town while attending school (Fig. 8.1) and parents may be away for months at a time tending cattle or visiting relatives in a distant homestead. During these long periods of separation, parents do not relinquish responsibility for the care of their children.

Because of the high frequencies of non-marital births and divorce (see Chapter 7), the biological parents of children often live in separate homesteads. If at least one of the biological parents claimed responsibility for the care of their children, we classified them as *not* fostered.

In the previous chapter, we described the Herero custom in which men purchase the patrilineal rights in the children that they have with unmarried girlfriends. When a man purchases rights in his children, they become his legal offspring and members of his homestead. Children who have already been fostered out by the time their father 'buys' them usually continue to stay with their foster parents. If the children have not already been fostered out, their father may take them to his own homestead and give them to his wife, his mother, or some other relative to raise. We always classified these children as fostered. Often, however, the children stay with their mother until they are old enough to look after themselves in their father's homestead. We classified these children as *not* fostered since either or both biological parents raised them.

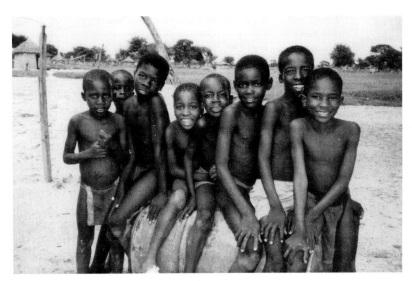

Fig. 8.1. Sehitwa school children. Many rural children are sent to live with relatives in towns where there are schools.

When couples divorce, women usually return to their own kinsmen. Since children that they had during their marriages legally belong to the homesteads of their husbands, many women leave behind their children. Those that are still young may be fostered out. Many other women, however, take their young children with them. We do not understand the politics of child custody after divorce. Our view was that women were forced to leave behind their children at divorce until one of our Herero friends criticized such scandalous behaviour in the wife of one of his relatives. 'What kind of mother', he said, 'could leave behind her children?'

The death of biological parents, especially unmarried mothers, may also cause children to be fostered. Our story about Freda in Chapter 2 illustrates this point nicely. Freda, who had never married, died suddenly leaving four children. One small child was given to Freda's sister and another to Freda's mother's family. Several months later the biological father of her two older daughters paid Freda's father several cattle and received patrilineal rights in these daughters. Although the daughters had already married by the time the transaction occurred, they became their biological father's legal offspring and became entitled to support from him.

Although the divorce or death of parents is the reason many children become fostered, the majority are fostered for less obvious reasons. Most children who are fostered are given to their foster parents by the time they

Table 8.1.   Ages at which children are fostered

Age	At risk	No. fostered	Percentage
0–2	1414	297	21
3–10	818	96	12
11–15	611	6	1
Unknown	—	154	—

are 2 years old, long before their parents die or divorce. Table 8.1 shows the number of individuals at risk of fosterage during three age classes and the number of those at risk who were fostered. To avoid over-estimating the proportions fostered by age due to censoring, only individuals old enough to survive each age class are counted. For example, only individuals at least 2 years old in 1987, the year before we began asking Herero about fosterage,[1] were included in the 0–2-year-old age class. The overall proportion of children fostered is under-estimated, however, since we excluded information about 154 individuals who were fostered out at unknown ages.

We chose wide age classes in Table 8.1 because many Herero did not recall the exact ages at which they or their children were fostered out. Most were able to provide at least a developmental stage for this event. We assigned developmental stages to one of the following age classes: (1) 0–2 years, (2) 3–10 years, and (3) 11–15 years. Herero most often told us that a child was fostered after it was weaned ('after breast'). Since Herero told us that they usually wean their children before they are two years old, we always scored this response in the first category (between 0 and 2 years). We also heard answers such as, 'when she was old enough to fetch water', or, 'when she was a young girl walking alone'. Many would also say, 'When he was this size', and then rotate their palm, perpendicular to the ground, into the sun. In these cases we usually estimated the age at fosterage by asking our respondents to point to a nearby child who was at the developmental stage they described and recorded that child's age for our answer.

Few children are fostered out during their first year of life and only under special circumstances. One young woman told us that she had fostered out her 7-month-old infant so that she could return to school. Another elderly lady told us that she took the new-born of a daughter who had already experienced two infant deaths, induced lactation, and raised the daughter's first living child. One young man we know was raised by his father's sister

---

[1] In analyses in previous chapters we have used 1986 as our last complete observation year. Since we began collecting data on fosterage in 1988, the second year of our study, we use 1987 as the last complete observation year.

after his mother died during his birth. His aunt induced lactation and later sent him to an American graduate school.

Why fosterage occurs

Why parents foster out their children

Although child fosterage is widespread (Goody 1973; Fiawoo 1978; Goody 1982; Goody 1984; Oppong 1989; Isiugo-Abanihe 1984; Frank 1987; Betzig 1988; Bledsoe and Isiugo-Abanihe 1989; Page 1989), its function in African societies is unclear. Among Herero, fosterage has been prevalent for at least a century. Vedder (1966*b*) observed fosterage at the turn of the century and speculated, at the suggestion of Herero, that fosterage was a form of 'child insurance'. Parents minimized their chances of losing all their children to epidemics by spreading them out among relatives.

We tried asking our Herero friends why they fostered out their children and got confused looks. After explaining to them that we have no similar custom in America, they became astounded. Their astonishment turned to horror when they learned that Americans allow perfect strangers to adopt their children. Unlike American and European adoption practices, Herero child fosterage occurs only between friends and relatives. Herero retain close ties with the children they foster out and say that they always keep an eye on them. Herero told us that they may retrieve that children they have fostered out at any time, but especially if they are being treated poorly. They may retrieve a child by going to him or her and asking, 'Child, where are your things?' If the situation is bad, they may just take the child home and buy him or her new things later.

Benefits

Economic opportunities   Other studies have attempted to understand child fosterage by examining economic aspects of fosterage, such as the economic costs and benefits of raising children (Turke 1989). Bledsoe and Isiugo-Abanihe (1989), following Goody (1982), distinguished between two types of foster children among the Mende of Sierra Leone, learning and household children and granny children. Learning and household children are fostered out so that the children may acquire some special training, such as schooling, while under the guardianship of the foster parent, who receives compensation. Granny foster parents take children at younger ages and often raise them until they are old enough to start school or other training. The granny may be the child's biological or classificatory grandmother or any older woman.

Fosterage among Herero is most similar to granny fosterage in the sense that foster parents act as child caretakers rather than providers of educational or other opportunities, and they are usually not compensated for their care. Herero children do stay with relatives (or non-relatives) while attending school in villages away from home, but Herero clearly distinguish these arrangements from fosterage. These children receive accommodation only: they are still dependent on another caretaker for economic support. Foster parents, however, usually provide support, such as clothing, food, fees, for the children they raise and, if they choose to send them to school, may arrange accommodation for them in another village. In a few cases, the child's natal homestead provided the accommodation.

As in the case of the Mende, Herero sometimes foster their children to wean them, and these children stay with foster parents for a few months or years only. Relationships between foster parents and the children they raise, especially girls, are usually less ephemeral. A foster daughter, especially if she is unmarried, will often give her own children to her foster parent. Before giving birth, a Herero woman customarily returns to her mother, who will assist her in childbirth and care for her and her new-born during the post-partum seclusion period (usually lasting about two months), but the 'mother' is often the foster mother rather than the biological mother. More often, however, children who have been fostered will return to their natal homestead late in their teens to help tend livestock if they are boys or to become engaged if they are girls.

Fosterage and fertility　Parents can benefit from fostering out their children in several ways. Mothers who are able to foster out their children may be able to wean them at earlier ages. By weaning children earlier, mothers may resume cycling sooner and become pregnant again sooner. Through fosterage, Herero women may reduce their birth intervals to achieve the high levels of fertility they desire. At the same time, mothers who are able to find others to raise some of their children for them save resources. The resources they save may allow them to either rear their other children more successfully or else produce more of them. For example, mothers who foster out children may be more capable of providing enough food for their other children or else keep a more watchful eye on them and better tend to them when they are ill. More food and better supervision may result in higher survival of their children. Since women who foster need to spend less time raising children, they have more time to spend pursuing mates or economic activities (Fig. 8.2).

From a simple Darwinian perspective, child fosterage is an attractive reproductive strategy for mothers. If fosterage allows women to increase their fertility without decreasing the survival of their children, then women who foster out their children will increase their genetic contribution to future generations. Below we examine the potential cost, in terms of child survival, associated with child fosterage. Later we discuss the other side of this issue: the biological cost to foster parents of rearing the offspring of

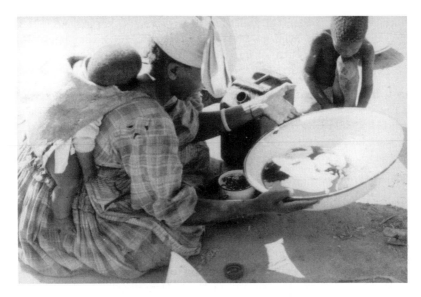

Fig. 8.2. Neighbor babysitting infant. It may be easier for Herero mothers to find foster parents than to find babysitters to look after their small children. The mother of the infant on this woman's back lives in a nearby homestead. She is away lifting water for goats. The babysitter is cooking *omaze* (see Fig. 1.8) and has an infant of her own.

others.

Costs

Parents who allow others to raise their children may incur a significant cost. Fostering may decrease child survival because children who have been fostered into a household often receive less care and fewer resources than children who are raised by their own parents. Among the Mende in Sierra Leone, for example, young fostered children appear to receive less medical care and more often suffered from malnutrition than non-fostered children (Bledsoe *et al.* 1988). These aspects of morbidity would lead to higher death rates among fostered children or to poorer reproductive prospects for them when they matured (Silk 1987; Bledsoe *et al.* 1988; Sudre *et al.* 1990).

We related earlier the concern Herero parents expressed to us regarding the welfare of children that they had fostered out. A few acknowledged that some of their children were well treated and educated by their foster parents but complained that other children were just made to work. Because most children are fostered out to the elderly (see below), few are in competition with the biological children of their foster parents but they may be in competition with other children living in the same homestead. Herero acknowledge the potential for favouritism and recognize that it may have serious consequences. One of our friends, who had been fostered out to a distant relative, related this story:

I was living in a village far from my mother. Then my uncle saw me. He saw that I was playing with the other children but that I did not look like them. I looked like a child who had no mother, no father, or any relative on earth. My uncle went back and told my mother. She came and got me and gave me to my uncle's mother. I stayed with her until she died.

Our friend told us that the food he was given during his stay with the first foster parent was of poor quality and that he was often sick with diarrhoea.

Another friend of ours related to us what often happens in these situations:

Say you send your child and the one you raise to fetch water. They take a long time so you beat the one you raise but not your own. Even food—your own child you give much food but the one you raise you give little food. When you buy clothes, you buy nice ones for your own child but not for the one you raise.

We hesitate to emphasize these negative aspects of child fosterage because we do not know how common poor treatment of foster children is, and it certainly was not condoned. 'This is not a good thing', we were told. 'If you give them food, you have to give them the same. It must be equal'. We saw many situations in which fostered in children were doted upon, and often these children had no kinship ties with the individuals raising them. One elderly couple we knew proudly gave us regular updates on the progress of a toddler they were raising for a woman from another tribe. This same couple had also taken in a strange homeless woman who appeared to be mentally unstable.

Since it is possible that Herero children who are fostered receive less parental care (i.e. less food or supervision) than children who are not fostered, we constructed life tables for the children we ascertained through parents and looked for differences in survival between Herero children who were fostered and those who were not. We used the Kaplan–Meier (product-limit) life table method described in previous chapters. Kaplan–Meier estimates produce life tables for censored data. If $F(t)$ is the survivorship function, n_j is the number at risk at time j, and d_j is the number of deaths occurring at time j, then the survivorship function can be estimated by (Kalbfleisch and Prentice 1980)

$$\hat{F}(t) = \prod_{j|t_j < t} \frac{n_j - d_j}{n_j}.$$

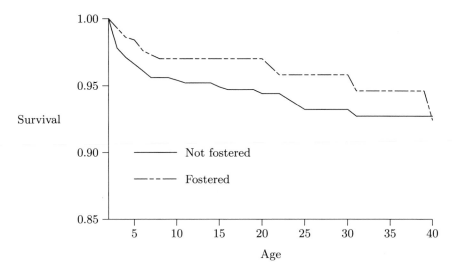

Fig. 8.3. Survivor curves for fostered and non-fostered children. The differences between the two curves are not statistically significant.

$\hat{F}(t)$ is thus the conditional probability of surviving.

Using the formula, we constructed separate survival curves for fostered and non-fostered children. They are shown in Fig. 8.3. The figure indicates that fostered children survive *better* than non-fostered children, but the differences are not statistically significant.[2] The curves show the survival experience of 1239 children who were at least 2 years old in 1985, 455 of whom were ever fostered out. We did not distinguish between the sexes because there were only 17 deaths among fostered children.

We began the survivor curves at age 2 because very few children are fostered at earlier ages. Including infants and 1-year-olds in the survivor curves increases the apparent protective effect of fosterage on survival. The slightly higher survival of fostered children is probably due to bias in the way we collected our data. Although the graph indicates that children who are fostered out survive better, it is also true that only children who survive can be fostered. For example, non-fostered children who die early in their third year of life are at risk of fosterage for only part of the year. In any case, the differences indicated by the graph are not statistically significant.

Based on our analysis, it appears that Herero children who are fostered out survive at least as well as children who are raised by their own parents. If fostered Herero children do receive less or possibly more care than non-

---

[2]We used the Mantel log-rank test available in the survival module of the PC version of SYSTAT to test whether the two curves represented identical survivor functions. The X^2 statistic was 1.69 with one degree of freedom, $p = 0.19$.

Table 8.2. Number of Herero who ever raised a foster child by their age in 1986. See text for details

| | Women | | | Men | | |
| | Fostered in children | | | Fostered in children | | |
Age	Y	N	Total	Y	N	Total
<=60	29	8	37	15	9	24
45–59	31	9	40	8	19	27
30–44	19	20	39	2	7	9
<30	6	69	75	0	7	7
Total	85	106	188	25	42	67

fostered children, the situation is not serious enough to result in a large mortality differential. Our sample is not large enough to detect subtle differences, however, and a proper analysis of the effect of fosterage on survival of children requires more careful control over the ages at which fosterage occurs. Unfortunately, most Herero were unable to provide us with this information about their children.

Why foster in

To get an alternative perspective on child fosterage, we tried asking Herero why they took in a foster child and got uniformative answers such as, 'because she is my daughter's child', 'because I wanted to help my son', or, 'because I quit giving birth'. Most of the Herero who foster in children were women past reproductive age, as shown in Table 8.2. The table shows the age distribution of 188 Herero women and 67 Herero men that we interviewed about foster parenting. Nearly 70 per cent of the post-reproductive women told us that they had taken in at least one foster child at some point in their life. Only 22 per cent of women less than 45 years old had taken in a foster child. The table shows comparable statistics for men, but we are reluctant to make much of them because of the way we recorded our data. Many married couples claimed that they both raised the same children. Since women do the child-rearing, we counted them, rather than their husbands, as the foster parent. Unfortunately, we did not ask all men if their wives helped raise the children they told us about. In the tabulations for men in the table, men were counted as foster parents either if they told us they raised a child or if one of their wives raised a child. The table indicates that women are more likely to take in foster children than men and at younger ages, but because of the way we tabulated our data these figures probably do not accurately reflect differences between the sexes. Still, the data for men indicate that foster parenting is more common among older Herero.

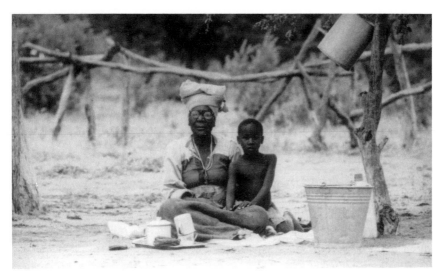

Fig. 8.4.   Old Herero woman with the young boy she raises.

Economic advantages

Because most foster parents are elderly, the children they raise may be a valued source of labour (Fig. 8.4). A few Herero told us that they like to take in foster children because the children can bring them tea in the morning while they are still sleeping, fetch water, milk cows, keep house, and look after livestock (Fig. 8.5). We pointed out to them that most children are so small when they are fostered out that it is several years before they are old enough to help their foster parents. By that time, many of them have enrolled in school and, as adults, leave their foster parents' homesteads. They also acknowledged that foster parents have to spend money on food, clothing, and schooling for children that they foster in. Some countered that they received a share of the bride-wealth for girls they helped raised. We do not believe that this compensation is sufficient motivation for rearing foster children. Bride-wealth is never more than three cattle. Foster parents are typically two generations older than the children they raise and have often passed away by the time their foster daughters marry. When pressed, many Herero were unsure whether the economic benefits of taking in foster children outweighed the costs. To those who liked to raise children, however, no cost seemed too great.

In sum, our view is that individuals do not increase their economic productivity by taking in foster children. The domestic tasks that girls perform could be done more cheaply by paying them piecemeal for their

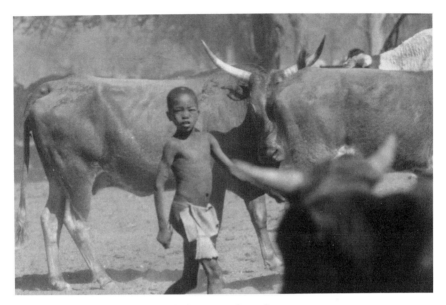

Fig. 8.5. Young Herero boy helping tend cattle.

work. Although boys do help tend livestock, herding is not as important to livestock management as it is among many East African pastoralists (Gulliver 1955; Vivelo 1977). A number of Herero families hire children from other ethnic groups to help tend their livestock (Fig. 8.6) while their own children attend school. Only one of the many women who reported that they were foster mothers claimed to receive economic support. This woman said that she was compensated with food by the biological parents of the child she was raising.

Biological costs and benefits

From a simple Darwinian perspective, natural selection should favour behaviours that cause individuals to leave more surviving offspring than others and the number of surviving offspring an individual leaves is often used as a proxy for Darwinian fitness. Since an individual shares identical copies of a fraction of his or her genes with relatives, individuals may increase their fitness by increasing the reproductive success of relatives. Because mothers who are able to foster out their children may increase their fertility by shortening their birth intervals, a grandmother can indirectly increase her own fitness by rearing her daughter's children.

From the same point of view, individuals who raise the children of others may seem to be behaving maladaptively (Silk 1987; Silk 1990). In terms of

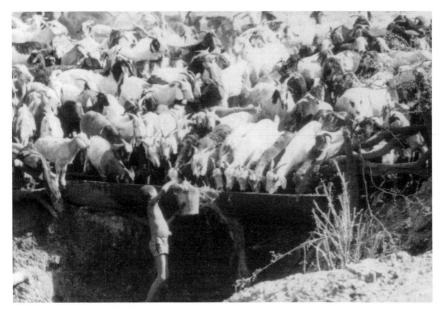

Fig. 8.6. Young Mbukushu boy watering Herero goats and sheep.

reproductive success, they are nurturing offspring whose genetic contribution to future generations is in competition with their own. For most of the Herero who were fostered out, we obtained the name of the foster parent. We also tried to elicit the biological relationship between the individual who was fostered and the person who was raising him or her. A tabulation of the relationship between children and their foster parent is shown in Table 8.3. The table must be interpreted cautiously. We are not sure we were always successful in our efforts to get Herero to distinguish between biological and classificatory relatives. We also collapsed both full- and half-siblings into the *sib* category. Because of the relative lack of paternity confidence and polygyny, individuals who said that they were related through male lineages or a parent's sibling were often not biologically related at all. We also have a large number of individuals classified as *unknown*. In most of these cases, we knew who the foster parent was, but we were not careful to ascertain the relationship between a child and the individual raising it. Since we always ascertained the names of the mother and father of the people we interviewed, we know that the majority of individuals in the *unknown* class were not raised by close relatives (i.e. they were not raised by a grandparent). With these limitations of the data in mind, we can still make use of our table. The table shows that 26 per cent (159/621)

Table 8.3. Putative relationship of children to their foster parents

	Mother's	Father's	Total
Mother/father/spouse	159	35	194
Sib	53	40	93
Mother's mother/father/sib	38	6	44
Father's mother/father/sib	17	1	18
Other relative	29	28	57
Sib			1
Not related			16
Unknown			198
Total	296	110	621

of children who are fostered are raised by maternal grandparents[3] while 6 per cent (35/621) are raised by paternal grandparents.[4] Another 15 per cent (93/621) are raised by a half or full sibling of their mother or father. One individual was raised by a sibling. The remainder of fostered children (54 per cent) were also raised by individuals who were genetically related to them by no more than 25 per cent. In sum, the table shows that many individuals are raised by close relatives, but that many more are not.

While it is hard to imagine people contemplating the pros and cons of fostering out their children and making decisions based on expected gains in Darwinian fitness, it is not so hard to imagine that behaviours detrimental to an individual's fitness will 'die out', be they genetic or cultural traits. Under simple genetic models of inheritance, genes coding for a behaviour should decrease in frequency if they reduce the fitness of their bearers. By analogy, a fitness-reducing behaviour that is culturally transmitted from parent to offspring should also decrease in frequency since it, too, will have fewer and fewer bearers in subsequent generations. On the other hand, it is possible for maladaptive culturally transmitted traits to persist (Boyd and Richerson 1985; Richerson and Boyd 1989; Rogers 1988). Some also argue that human behaviour ought to be understood through examination of psychological underpinnings (Symons 1989). For example, child fosterage in Africa may be an adaptation to a past social environment, such as one with chronic warfare or some other condition not present today.

---

[3]That is, they are being raised by either their mother's mother, their mother's father, or a spouse of one of these grandparents (mother's mother's spouse or mother's father's spouse).

[4]That is, they are being raised by either their father's mother, their father's father, or a spouse of one of these grandparents (father's mother's spouse or father's father's spouse).

A test of ideas

We have considered the costs and benefits of fosterage. We suggested that women may be motivated to foster out their children because of gains in reproductive success. We have also argued that reproductive gains to mothers who foster out result in costs to foster parents who are not closely related to the children they raise. We also discussed economic reasons why Herero may foster in or foster out children. We believe that Herero children do not work enough for their foster parents to offset the cost of raising them. If we are wrong, we wonder why biological parents would give away such valuable economic commodities. There are certainly a number of issues involved that we do not understand, and we emphasize that rights in and obligations to children probably extend throughout the kin networks of both biological and foster parents of children. Central to our understanding of child fosterage then is the direction of liability involved in the exhange of children. In other words, are individuals getting or giving a favour by fostering children?

Herero were poor informants about why they foster in or foster out children, but we can get at the issue of whether fostering is regulated by supply of vs demand for foster children in other ways. In Chapter 3 we observed a high sex mortality differential among Herero children that suggests a strong preference for female children. If fostering is driven by 'demand' for children by foster parents who take children from their mothers, then the apparent sex preference for female children should result in more female children being fostered out than male. Alternatively, if fostering is driven by 'supply' of children, we expect that Herero mothers slough the least desired sex, resulting in more male children being fostered out than female.

In Chapter 7 we discussed in detail alternative life course strategies for the sexes. We emphasized the male focus on social reproduction and the female focus on biological reproduction. We suggested that men delay arranging marriages for their daughters so that the daughters will produce a few children for their own patrilineages. Once their daughters marry, the children they subsequently bear belong to the patrilineages of their husbands. Based on our scenario, we expect to find that the children that women bear before they marry are fostered out more than children that they have during their marriages. The children of unmarried mothers are fostered out more because their mothers' fathers (who have the patrilineal rights in them) want them, while the children of married mothers are fostered less because their own fathers are entitled to them.[5]

---

[5] Previously we believed that the children of unmarried mothers would be fostered more because their mothers were not allowed to bring them to their husbands' homesteads. We discuss this alternative interpretation later.

Below we examine these ideas using log-linear models that quantify the relationship between Herero child fosterage rates and the sex of children and the marital status of mothers. We also look for associations between several measures of female reproductive rates and fosterage. If fosterage is sensitive to the fertility of women, fosterage rates should have increased in the 1960s in response to the dramatic increase in female fertility described in Chapter 5. Similarly, we expect that fosterage rates should respond to changes in female reproductive rates associated with the ageing of women during their reproductive spans. We outline these expectations in more detail later.

Results

Log-linear models

Log-linear modelling is a method for analysing multi-way contingency tables in which cell frequencies are estimated with a model in which interaction between variables is specified (Fienberg 1980). A model's goodness of fit can be tested by computing either the likelihood ratio, G^2, or Pearson's chi-square statistic, X^2, both of which approximate χ^2 distributions for large samples when the model fitted is correct (Fienberg 1980). The degrees of freedom associated with each statistic are equal to the number of cells in the table less the number of parameters fitted. Since the G^2 statistics can be partitioned to test nested models, we report them rather than X^2 statistics. We used the program BMDP, PF4, to fit log-linear models in this chapter.

The simplest log-linear model is the model of independence for a two-by-two contingency table in which interaction between rows and columns is assumed to be zero. The log-linear equation for Table 3.3 is given by

$$\ln(F_{ij}) = \theta + \lambda_i^{\mathrm{M}} + \lambda_j^{\mathrm{S}}, \quad \lambda_{ij}^{\mathrm{MS}} = 0,$$

where $\ln(F_{ij})$ is the natural log of the expected frequency of the cell in the ith row and jth column, θ is the grand mean, λ_i^{M} is the row effect, or the deviation from the mean due to mortality, λ_j^{S} is the column effect, or deviation from the mean due to sex, and $\lambda_{ij}^{\mathrm{MS}}$ is the effect of interaction between the rows and columns. Since the X^2 statistic for this model is large relative to its degrees of freedom (30.7, 1 d.f.), we reject the model of independence (that $\lambda^{\mathrm{MS}} = 0$). The alternative model is the saturated model, which in general includes effects for all possible interactions between all variables. A saturated model always fits the data perfectly but, since it has no degrees of freedom, its goodness of fit is not testable. Following convention, and for clarity of interpretation, all log-linear models in this chapter are hierarchical, meaning that any model that includes higher-ordered terms must also include all related lower-ordered terms. For example, a model that includes

λ^{MS} must also include λ^M and λ^S. Consequently, for ease of notation, a model in which lower ordered terms are zero implies that related higher ordered terms are also zero. For example, the model in which λ^M is zero implies that λ^{MS} is also zero.

Sources of bias

We described above how we collected our fostering data. This type of sampling can be biased in several ways. First, young children who were not fostered when we interviewed their parents are censored because they may still be fostered in future years. As a result, fostering rates of recently born individuals are low due to censoring rather than actual decline. Since only a small fraction of children are fostered out after age 10 (Table 8.1), bias due to censoring is probably negligible if we exclude children aged 10 years and younger from our log-linear analysis. We excluded 578 children who were born in or after 1977 from our analysis; of these, 185 (32 per cent) had already been fostered.

Similarly, non-fostered children who died are censored because they might have been fostered had they lived. Mortality can also cause ascertainment bias since we self-ascertained only individuals who survived to adulthood. For example, if fostered out children have higher mortality than non-fostered children, self-ascertained rates of fosterage will be lower than parent-ascertained rates. However, we detected no significant differences in survival between fostered and non-fostered children (Fig. 8.3). Since we cannot detect differences in mortality between fostered and non-fostered children, differential mortality is probably not an important source of ascertainment bias. In other words, self-ascertained individuals are probably not providing information about fosterage that is different from individuals who did not survive to self-report whether they were fostered. Since fosterage and a child's risk of death appear to be unrelated, to minimize bias due to censoring associated with mortality, we excluded 166 children (152 not fostered, 14 fostered) who died before age 10. Of these, 49 (46 not fostered, 3 fostered) children were also born after 1977.

Method of ascertainment can also bias interpretation of results if self-reported rates differ from parent-reported rates. In particular, very young children are parent-ascertained only, while very old individuals cannot be parent-ascertained. Since temporal trends in fosterage practices are of interest in this chapter, it is important to account for variation attributable to method of ascertainment.

Data based on memory recall can be biased since events that happened long ago are more likely to be forgotten than events that occur more recently. In the case of fosterage, parents may 'forget' that they fostered their children, especially since many children eventually return to their natal homesteads. In contrast, an individual is less likely to 'forget' that he or she was fostered since fosterage constitutes a major event in an individual's life, more so than the parent's. If temporal variation in fostering is biased by forgetting, the proportion of children fostered will appear to increase through time, but, due to differential recall between individuals and parents, rates based on parent-ascertained data should increase more rapidly than those self-ascertained.

To assess the relationship between ascertainment method and fosterage, we categorized the data in Table 8.4 by a child's ascertainment (A), sex (S), birth cohort (C), and fostering status (F). Since more females were self-ascertained than males, we added sex as a variable because females are consistently fostered at a higher rate than males (see below). In general, 42 per cent of all females are fostered compared to about 30 per cent of males. We excluded children in the cohort 1968–77 (352 cases) to avoid 0 counts in the self-ascertained cells; we excluded 24 additional children because their birth years were unknown. The log-linear model

$$\ln(F) = \theta + \lambda^A + \lambda^S + \lambda^C + \lambda^F + \lambda^{AS} + \lambda^{AC} + \lambda^{SC} + \lambda^{SF} + \lambda^{CF}, \quad \lambda^{AF} = 0,$$

was fit to these data. This log-linear model is similar to the logit model in which fostering is the response variable and ascertainment, sex, and birth cohort are the predictor variables (Fienberg 1980). Terms specifying interaction between the predictor variables do not appear in first-order logit models, and they are not of interest here either. Restricting attention to interaction between fosterage and the predictor variables, the model above says that a child's sex and birth cohort affects his (or her) chances of being fostered out, but, because λ^{AF} is assumed to be zero, how the child was ascertained does not affect fosterage response. The G^2 of 8.79 (14 d.f., $p = 0.84$) for this model indicates a good fit to the data. Including a term for interaction between fosterage and ascertainment method ($\lambda^{AF} \neq 0$) results in a smaller G^2 of 8.00 but with only one less degree of freedom. Since the G^2 for the nested comparison of the two models is 0.79 (1 d.f., $p > 0.25$), we cannot reject the hypothesis that $\lambda^{AF} = 0$.

The results of this analysis indicate that fosterage is independent of ascertainment method and that temporal variation in fostering rates is not attributable to method of ascertainment. Furthermore, there is no evidence to support the hypothesis that individuals 'forget' they or their children were fostered, since fosterage that occurred long ago is equally remembered by both parents and children. Since ascertainment method appears to be independent of reporting of fosterage, the contingency table can be collapsed over this variable (Fienberg 1980) when the logit model analogue is used. Consequently, data obtained using both ascertainment methods were pooled in the analyses below.

Table 8.4. Ascertainment, fosterage, sex and birth cohort

Asc.	Fost.	Sex	Cohort ≤1937	1938–1947	1948–1957	1958–1967	Total
P	N	F	10	26	37	62	135
		M	25	35	39	65	164
	Y	F	7	15	25	53	100
		M	6	14	16	35	71
S	N	F	84	36	36	38	194
		M	69	19	6	10	104
	Y	F	40	25	25	49	139
		M	12	6	5	8	31
Total			253	176	189	320	938

Characteristics of fostered children

We showed in Chapter 5 that fertility rates have been increasing in this century. Similarly, fostering rates have increased through time. Fig. 8.7 is a graph of fostering rates plotted by child's birth year for children born to parents who married each other and to parents who did not marry each other. We considered a child's parents to be married to each other if at any time before or subsequent to the child's birth the child's mother and putative father were wed to each other. We classified a child as a child of unmarried parents if the child's mother and putative father were never married to each other, although they may have been married to someone else at some point in their life cycle. Thus, there can be two kinds of 'unmarried parents'— those that *ever marry* and those that *never marry*; this distinction will be important later. Occasionally, women named deceased husbands as fathers, which according to Herero custom means that the child belongs to the husband's patrilineage; in these cases we considered the child's parents to be unmarried.

We smoothed the curves in Fig. 8.7 to reduce noise in the rates from data sparseness. The *parents married* curve shows a wave with a period of about 10 years. We have fewer data to construct the *parents unmarried* curve, especially before 1940 when we begin the curve, but the *parents unmarried* curve has the same wave apparent in the *parents married* curve. We show in Chapter 10 that a wave in the population pyramid has persisted throughout this century, with pinches occurring about every 20 years (see Fig. 10.4). It is possible that the wave in the curves in Fig. 8.7 is caused by fluctuations in the supply of foster children or, conversely, in the supply of foster parents produced by the wave in the population pyramid. The population pyramid wave affects the proportion of children to adults. Overall, the figure shows that fostering rates have increased through time and that

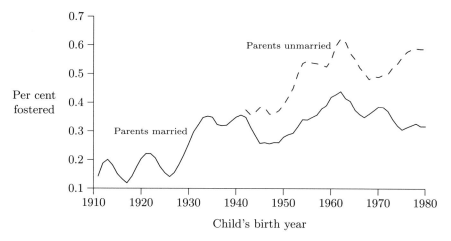

Fig. 8.7. Fostering rates by parent's marital status. The proportion of children of unmarried parents fostered before 1940 is not shown due to data sparseness. The rates were smoothed using 5-year running averages and resmoothed using 3-year running averages.

children of unmarried parents appear to be fostered out at a higher rate than children of married parents.

Table 8.5 is a tabulation of the number of children fostered by sex, child's birth cohort, and parent's marital status. We fit a log-linear model to these data to assess the effects of sex (S), child's birth cohort (C), and parent's marital status (P) on fosterage (F). This analysis excluded 33 children because either their parent's marital status (9 cases) or year of birth (24 cases) was unknown. Although we are interested in the effect of mother's age on risk of fosterage, we examine this separately below because of the pattern in the data.

The model

$$\ln(F) = \theta + \lambda^{S} + \lambda^{F} + \lambda^{C} + \lambda^{P} + \lambda^{SF} + \lambda^{CF} + \lambda^{PF} + \lambda^{CP}, \quad \lambda^{SC} = \lambda^{SP} = 0,$$

provides an adequate fit to the data ($G^2 = 25.02$, 22 d.f., $p = 0.2962$). The estimates of the parameters and their standard errors for the interactions between the predictor variables of interest (cohort, parent's marital status, and sex) and fosterage (the response variable) are given in Table 8.6. Following Clogg and Eliason (1987), we converted the estimates of the λ's to odds ratios.

Odds ratios are measures of association in two-by-two tables (or in two-by-two subtables) with values ranging between 0 and ∞. An odds ratio of 1 means that the probabilities of association are equal. Odds ratios less than 1 indicate a negative association between the variables while odds ratios

Table 8.5. Fosterage, sex, parent's marital status, and birth cohort. PM is parents married

			Cohort					
				1938–	1948–	1958–	1968–	
Fost.	Sex	PM	≤1937	1947	1957	1967	1977	Total
N	F	N	6	12	16	25	19	78
		Y	81	39	40	59	69	288
	M	N	9	9	13	13	25	69
		Y	71	38	30	60	77	276
Y	F	N	5	6	16	26	27	80
		Y	34	24	25	55	51	189
	M	N	5	5	10	17	30	67
		Y	11	9	10	23	25	78
Total			222	142	160	278	323	1125

Table 8.6. Effects of cohort, parent's marital status, and sex on fosterage Model fitted is $\ln(F) = \theta + \lambda^S + \lambda^F + \lambda^P + \lambda^C + \lambda^{SF} + \lambda^{PF} + \lambda^{CF} + \lambda^{CP}$, $\lambda^{SC} = \lambda^{SP} = 0$. $G^2 = 25.02$, 22 d.f., $p = 0.296$. Partial associations are $G^2(\lambda^{CF}) = 18.11$, 4 d.f., $G^2(\lambda^{PF}) = 23.95$, 4 d.f. and $G^2(\lambda^{SF}) = 22.31$, 1 d.f. All probabilities for the partial associations are less than 0.001

Effects		Parameter	Standard error	Odds ratio
λ^{CF}	Before 1938	−0.207	0.070	0.48
	1938–1947	−0.091	0.079	0.60
	1948–1957	0.030	0.073	0.77
	1958–1967	0.162	0.058	1.00
	1968–1977	0.106	0.056	0.89
λ^{PF}	Parents not married	0.166	0.035	1.94
λ^{SF}	Female	0.140	0.032	1.75

greater than 1 indicate positive association. For the cohort effect, we use the cohort 1958–67 (about when fertility began increasing) as a reference cohort to which the probability of being fostered is compared. The increase in the odds ratios up until the reference period means that the odds of being fostered for children born during these periods has increased relative to the odds of being fostered for children born between 1958 and 1967. In particular, children born before 1938 are about half (0.48 times) as likely to be fostered as children born in the reference period. The risk of fosterage, relative to the reference period, declines among children in the last cohort who are 0.89 times as likely to be fostered as children belonging to the reference cohort.

The odds ratio of 1.94 for the effect of parent's marital status on fosterage means that children of unmarried parents are nearly two times as likely to be fostered as children of married parents. Similarly, female children are 1.75 times more likely to be fostered than male children.

The significance of the effects of the predictor variables of interest on fosterage can be tested by examining the partial association of these variables. They are included in Table 8.6. All probabilities are 0.001 or less, indicating that their effect on fosterage is highly significant.

Fosterage and mother's age

While the level of fertility varies between and within populations through time, the age pattern of marital fertility in non-contracepting populations generally does not (Henry 1961; Wood 1989). Similarly, the age-specific fertility rates for Herero summarized above from Chapter 5 show that the level of fertility has increased through time and that fertility is always highest among women aged 20–4. In general, age-specific marital fertility rates in natural fertility populations increase rapidly as girls become reproductively mature in their teens, peaking in the mid-20s, after which age-specific fertility rates decline gradually towards zero as women approach menopause.

Fosterage can increase fertility by causing children to be weaned earlier, thereby removing the contraceptive effects of lactation. Consequently, fosterage may reduce the length of birth intervals by allowing mothers who foster their children to reconceive sooner so that they are able to fit more births into their reproductive span. Fosterage may also be a result rather than a cause of high fertility and short birth intervals, since a mother who becomes pregnant while still breast-feeding the previous born offspring may be more inclined to foster out the child; several Herero reported independently that they considered the breast-milk of a pregnant woman harmful to the nursling and that these children should be weaned. Since fertility is highest, and therefore birth intervals shortest, among women in their early 20s, mothers who are fostering children in response to the length of birth intervals should be fostering more of their children early in reproduction and fewer of them later.

The reproductive potential of a woman, or the number of children she can expect to have in the future, may also underlie motivation for fosterage. In general, a woman's reproductive potential is at a maximum before the beginning of reproduction and declines from then on due to age-related increases in fetal mortality and decreases in fecundity. If women are fostering their children in anticipation of future reproductive output, fostering rates should also decline with a woman's age. In other words, if fosterage saves women reproductive effort that they can instead use to produce additional offspring, it has potentially the greatest effect early in reproduction since there is no point in reserving parental investment for future offspring that are unlikely to be born.

A model developed by Pennington and Harpending (1988) would also predict a decline in fosterage rates with maternal age for similar reasons. This model weighs the relative importance of environmental factors and parental care on child survival in varying ecological settings and predicts, all other factors being equal, that women should invest longer intervals of care in children that they bear, e.g. through lactation, as their fertility declines. Under the assumptions of this model, mothers maximize their reproductive success by nurturing later born offspring more intensely when increases in parental care enhance the child's survival. Since fosterage frequently severs parental investment at weaning, the Pennington and Harpending model suggests that Herero mothers would do better by investing more heavily in later born offspring than by fostering them out, providing that this extra investment increased the survival of the offspring.

If women are fostering their children in response to the number of births they have already had, then older mothers would also be expected to foster out more of their children than younger mothers due to the correlation between parity and maternal age. That is, most women having a first birth are younger than women having higher-ordered births, and only older women have had a chance to have many births. We do not directly test the relationship between parity and fosterage because we do not know the parity of the mothers of the individuals in our sample who were self-ascertained. Also, the mothers in the sample are at various points in their reproductive span so that we can measure the correlation between the completed number of births to women and the number of children that they fostered out for of only a small sample. The fact that many women have both marital and non-marital births makes analysis of the relationship between parity and fosterage even more difficult. Consequently, an obvious way to test the relationship between fosterage and fertility is not suitable at all.

A plot of fostering rates by mother's age for children whose parents are married and children whose parents are unmarried is shown in Fig. 8.8. We separated the data for children of unmarried parents into two curves to show differences in risk of fosterage between children whose mothers *never* married and children whose mothers *ever* married. We classified a mother as ever married if she had been married prior to a child's birth or married later, although she was never married to the father of the child (see clarification above). Most women marry at least once in life, but Herero marriage is very unstable (Chapter 7) so that many women marry several times during their reproductive span. It is not uncommon for a woman to have one or two births before her first marriage or to reproduce after becoming divorced or widowed, as there is no stigma attached to children born to unmarried women.

We constructed the separate curves for children of unmarried parents

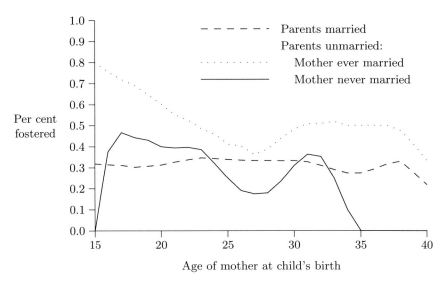

Fig. 8.8. Fostering rates by mother's marital status and age at birth. The rates were smoothed using 5-year running averages and resmoothed using 3-year running averages.

because of expected differences in risk of fosterage between children in these two categories. At marriage, most women leave their non-marital children with their father (i.e. the maternal grandfather of the children) so that marriage causes fosterage. The curve for 'ever married' mothers is higher than the curve for 'never married' mothers, indicating that these children are indeed at a higher risk of being fostered. Both curves show a tendency for fostering rates to decline from age 15 to the mid- to late 20s and then to increase. The differences in fostering rates of children of unmarried parents (mothers ever and never married combined) as given in Table 8.7 are statistically significant but do not correspond to any pattern expected to be associated with fertility. That both curves show the same pattern, however, suggests that the pattern is real. In contrast, this figure indicates that the children of married parents are at constant risk of being fostered regardless of their mothers' ages. Because fosterage does not increase during the peak reproductive years of women, these results suggest that there is no correlation between the length of birth intervals and fosterage. There is also no increase in the rate at which children born to older women are fostered, indicating that higher parity women do not foster more of their children than lower parity women.

Table 8.7. Effect of mother's age on fosterage for children whose parents did not marry each other. $X^2 = 21.594$, 4 d.f. Odds ratios are computed relative to the oldest category of mothers (mothers older than 34)

Mother's age	Fostered	Not fostered	Odds ratio
<20	60	29	5.02
20–24	41	42	2.37
25–29	12	28	1.04
30–34	13	10	3.16
>34	7	17	1.00

Discussion

Our log-linear analysis examining the association between fostering and temporal changes in fertility, sex of children, and the marital status of mothers appears contradictory. We found that female children are fostered out 1.75 times as often as male children and that the children of unmarried mothers are fostered out 1.94 times as often the children of married mothers, supporting the notion that fosterage is driven by demand for foster children. In contrast, we found that fosterage rates have doubled in this century, supporting the notion that fosterage is driven by supply of foster children. However, in a separate analysis, we examined the relationship between fostering rates and the age pattern of female fertility and found no support for the idea that women foster their children in response to their fertility.

Sex preferences for foster children

Herero do not express either behaviourally or verbally an obvious preference for children of any particular sex. The most overt expression we ever heard was from a Herero woman raising several of her son's children who told us she prefers fostering in girls because they help her, while boys help the men. In Chapter 3 we noted a huge sex differential in mortality, with girls surviving two to three times better than boys. Sex differentials of this magnitude are unusual and suggest a strong preference among Herero for female children. We suggested earlier in this chapter that this apparent sex preference for girls should give us insight into whether demand vs supply of children regulates fosterage. Since females are the preferred sex, we expect girls to be preferentially 'kept' by their mothers if mothers are in control of fosterage whereas girls would be preferentially 'taken' by foster parents if foster parents are in control. That girls are 1.75 times more likely to be fostered indicates that foster parents 'take' children from their biological parents rather than children being 'cast off' by biological parents onto foster parents.

Fostering and parents marital status

Unmarried women foster out children at nearly double the rate of married women—50 per cent of all children born to unmarried parents are fostered compared to 32 per cent of the children of married parents. We expected this finding because we noticed that children that women had before marriage seemed to be fostered before they married. Previously we believed that non-marital children were fostered out by women before they married because women were not allowed to bring the children they had with other men to their husbands' homesteads. In retrospect, this view contradicts what we knew about Herero. Since men seem to consider the children that their wives have with other men as boons to their lineages (see Chapters 1 and 7), it now seems more plausible that the children of an unmarried woman are fostered more because the new husband is not entitled to them. Instead, children are fostered more to other, more deserving relatives.

Our newer interpretation of the observation that children of unmarried women are fostered more than the children of married women is also more harmonious with the ideas we have developed in this volume regarding the concern of men with social rather than biological reproduction. Our observation is that the children of unmarried women who never eventually marry (and therefore would not be forced to foster out their non-marital children before moving to their husbands' homesteads) are still fostered much more often (46 per cent) than the children of married parents (32 per cent). Clearly there is some other reason why children are 'taken' from their biological mother. We suggest the reason is that the fathers of unmarried women delay marrying off their daughters so that their daughters will provide children for their own lineages. Fathers either keep their daughters' children in their own homesteads or foster them out to other relatives.

We can test our hypothesis by examining the relationship between a child's risk of being fostered and the survival of the child's maternal grandfather. If men delay marrying off their daughters so that the daughters will provide children for them, then only those men who are alive when their grandchildren are born can influence the rearing of them. We should find that the children of unmarried women are fostered more if their maternal grandfather is alive than if he is deceased. We find very strong support for our hypothesis in Table 8.8.

The table shows a cross-tabulation of the numbers of children fostered by the survival of their maternal grandfather. We categorized grandfathers who died before our study as deceased only if they died before the birth year of a child. We classified them as living if they died after the child was born. We were unable to determine for 507 children whether their maternal grandfathers died before or after they were born.

Table 8.8. Number of children fostered by survival of mother's father and by parent's marital status. X^2 for the contingency table in Part A is 0.32, 1 d.f., not significant. X^2 for the contingency table in Part B is 7.79, 1 d.f., $p \approx 0.005$

Part A: Parents married

		Mother's father dead		
		N	Y	Total
Fostered	N	163	106	274
	Y	89	65	154
Total		252	171	425

Part B: Parents not married

		Mother's father dead		
		N	Y	Total
Fostered	N	44	46	90
	Y	72	33	105
Total		116	79	195

The table shows that children whose parents are not married (Part B) have a 62 per cent chance of being fostered if their maternal grandfather is alive, but if their grandfather is dead their risk is only 42 per cent. The X^2 statistic for the cross-tabulation is 7.79 on one degree of freedom, having a probability of only about 0.005. The survival of the maternal grandfather has no effect at all on the chances that children born to married parents become fostered. Children born to married parents have a 35 per cent chance of being fostered if their maternal grandfathers are alive, compared to a 38 per cent chance if their maternal grandfathers are deceased. This difference is not statistically significant, and it is only slightly lower than the risk to children with deceased grandfathers born to unmarried parents. Table 8.8 strongly supports our notion that daughters have a reproductive role in their fathers' households.

Fostering and fertility

A closer look at the correspondence between temporal increases in fostering rates and fertility during the last few decades indicates that the impression that fosterage increased with fertility may be spurious. Our estimates of period fertility (Tables 5.1 and 5.2) indicate that fertility was uniformly low in the first half of the century and that it has been increasing since 1957–66. Our log-linear model indicates that fosterage rates were increasing in the decades before this period and that fosterage rates in fact declined in the 10-year-period (1968–77) following the fertility increase.

We also studied the correspondence between variation in fostering rates and the age pattern of female fertility. We found that the children of married parents are fostered out at a constant rate, regardless of their mothers' ages. The chances that children of unmarried parents get fostered out seem to vary with mothers' ages, but in a way that does not correspond to variation in age-related levels of fertility. Children born to women in their late 20s are least likely to be fostered out. Since we expected that women would foster more of their children during their peak reproductive years in the mid-20s, that women are fostering few of their children during this period is a strong indicator that, contrary to our hypothesis, women do not foster out their children in response to their fertility.

Conclusion

Our two examinations of an association between fostering and fertility provide very weak support for the idea that fosterage is regulated by women trying to foster out their children to increase their fertility or to get help from relatives because they have too many children to rear. Our other findings, the sex preference for female children and that the children of unmarried mothers are fostered out more than the children of married mothers, suggest that children are fostered out because foster parents take them from their biological parents. The apparent temporal increase in fosterage rates and the subsequent decline in this century may be due to the unusual age structure of the population in the early part of this century. We show in Chapter 10 that the founding Herero population in Botswana at the turn of the century consisted of a large proportion of young adults. Because of the low fertility, the maturation of the population produced a narrow population pyramid so that the ratio of young people to old people was increasing for several decades. Fosterage rates may have increased because there were more adults demanding foster children. The foster-child market may have been saturated by the increase in fertility in 1957–66, resulting in the subsequent decline in fosterage rates after 1967. Although these ideas have yet to be tested, Fig. 8.7, which indicates periodic fluctuations in fosterage rates, lends tentative support for them.

We also used our fosterage data to test the hypothesis that men delay marrying their daughters so that their daughters will produce children for their own lineages. We found that the children of unmarried women are much more likely to be fostered out if their maternal grandfathers were alive when they were born than if their grandfathers were deceased. We observed no similar effect for children born to married couples. These findings suggest that many women play important reproductive roles in their fathers' households. A large proportion of the children they bear (62 per cent) are taken from them and are either reared by their father or given to others. Although we do not fully understand why Herero like to take in foster children, they are clearly important assets.

9
Herero and !Kung comparative demography

Introduction

In the last two decades anthropologists have become increasingly interested in the possibility that variability in caloric intake and energy expenditure affect fertility. Much of the impetus for this interest was the finding that !Kung Bushmen, hunting and gathering people who occupy the same valleys of north-western Ngamiland as Herero, had low completed family sizes of four to five live births. The low fertility of the !Kung became incorporated into an anthropological legend about Bushmen—that they were affluent, cheerful, and gentle people who ate a lot of high fibre natural foods, lactated a long time, and got a lot of exercise (Sahlins 1968; Kolata 1974). This way of life led to 'natural' fertility control, according to the ideology, so that they had near zero population growth and were in long term balance with their environment. The natural state was lost when Herero and other pastoralists moved into their range. !Kung settled with Herero, began drinking milk and eating grain, quit walking long distances to forage, and their fertility increased dramatically through shorter birth intervals.

In this chapter we re-examine the foundation of this legend by comparing !Kung demography with that of the Herero. Since we know that the main Herero movement into the !Kung range occurred in the 1950s, we look at temporal changes in !Kung rates documented by Howell (1979) to understand how the arrival of the Herero changed the conditions of !Kung survival and reproduction.

Our interpretation of the !Kung data contradicts the legend. We will show that the arrival of Herero and their cattle led to a drastic decline in childhood mortality among the !Kung, probably because the milk from Herero cattle was available to !Kung children. There is no evidence that the new food source affected !Kung fertility. We argue that low !Kung fertility resulted from infectious agents rather than from long birth intervals and that food has a more important effect on mortality than on fertility.

The general idea in cultural ecology and in zoology about the link between food and fertility is that low fertility is a response to scarce resources. Both behavioural and biological mechanisms of regulation have been proposed. Behaviourally, individuals may achieve lower fertility by marrying late to reduce the effective length of the reproductive span or by breast-feeding for a long time to increase the spacing between births. Biologically, low caloric intakes or high activity levels may impair reproductive functioning by delaying reproductive maturity or by causing ovulatory failure (Frisch and McArthur 1974; Bentley 1985; Ellison 1990).Bentley, G. Permutations and combinations of these ideas are easy to find.

Generalizing from the !Kung, many human ecologists have come to believe that foraging populations adapt to low energy environments by regulating their fertility at low levels (Dumond 1975) and by investing a lot in each offspring. The Darwinian fitness of individuals is the result of compromises between extreme reproductive strategies in which parents invest heavily in a few children that survive well vs strategies in which parents invest less in more children that die at a higher rate (Pennington and Harpending 1988). !Kung were thought to maximize the number of offspring that survived by having small families. Although a number of interesting hypotheses have been proposed to explain how and why foraging populations have low fertility, empirical support for an association between subsistence mode and fertility is weak to non-existent (Campbell and Wood 1988). The underlying premise that !Kung had low reproductive rates because they were foragers has never been established.

Background

The !Kung belong to a larger group of Khoisan speakers who are believed to have subsisted in Southern Africa as hunter-gatherers for at least the last 24 000 years (Brooks 1989). At the time of European contact, the !Kung ranged in north-western Botswana, Namibia, and southern Angola. Group movement was seasonal, depending on the distribution of water and the availability of bush foods and game. At the end of the dry season, most congregated at a few permanent water holes but moved in smaller groups during the rainy season. There is a rich ethnographic literature about the !Kung, most of it the result of field-work by the Marshall family (Marshall 1976) and by investigators associated with the Harvard Kalahari Project summarized in Lee and DeVore (1976) and Lee (1979).

One of the notable findings of the Harvard Kalahari Project was that !Kung appeared to be characterized by unusual demographic rates. They had unusually low fertility and, in 1963–73, unexpectedly low mortality. These findings generated other research with aims of understanding the hunter-gatherer demographic adaptation. It was assumed that the conditions of foraging—mobility and the demands of infant carrying, low calorie availability, lack of soft weaning foods, long lactation—were the causes of the low fertility.

In the 1920s, Herero, as well as members of other Bantu groups in

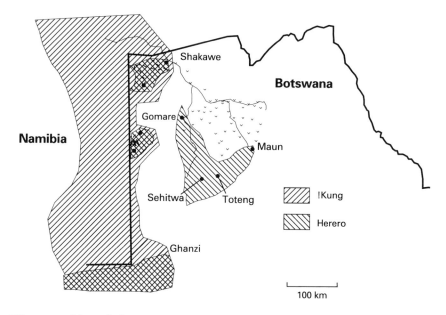

Fig. 9.1. Map of places in western Ngamiland occupied by !Kung and Herero.

Botswana, began expanding north-west into the Dobe, Xai Xai, NxauNxau, and Xaudum areas (see Fig. 1.2) previously occupied almost exclusively by !Kung (Howell 1979; Lee 1979; Solway and Lee 1990). Contact between Herero and !Kung accelerated in the 1950s when many more Herero moved into these areas following tsetse fly outbreaks near the Okavango Delta (Lee 1979; Howell 1979). Many !Kung, attracted by employment opportunities and more plentiful food, settled at the Herero homesteads. The areas presently occupied by Herero and !Kung are shown in Fig. 9.1.

The western expansion of pastoralists from the Okavango Delta into north-western Ngamiland originally extended beyond the Botswana border into Namibia. However, in 1957 the police shot many of their cattle and forced the Herero and other Bantu back into Botswana. This year became known in the Herero calendar as *ombura ojozongombe za Tsumkwe*, the year the cattle were shot at Tsumkwe.

Today there are probably less than 2000 !Kung living in Botswana. Many who lived north of the Qangwa valley in 1967 now reside in Namibia. In Chapter 10, we estimated that there were 10 000–15 000 Herero in Botswana in 1986. Together these populations represent about one-quarter of the population of Ngamiland and 2 per cent of the population of Botswana. For various reasons, few !Kung, if any, presently hunt and gather full-time. Many raise livestock of their own, but more are employed by Herero either as herders or casual labourers.

Sources of data

Most of the !Kung data that we use in this chapter are taken from Howell (1979), whose study took place in the Dobe region. !Kung did not know their years of birth so Howell estimated them by age-ranking individuals and then assuming that the proportions of population at each age fit a stable age distribution. Although Howell's method was suitable for comparisons within the !Kung population, the age estimates of some !Kung may be inaccurate if the assumption that the !Kung population was stable is inappropriate or if Howell chose the wrong stable age distribution. On the other hand, she was able to obtain exact ages of children born in 1963–73. Her population consisted of over 500 !Kung who had lived in the Dobe region during her study.

We also use the results of the larger but less detailed demographic survey of !Kung conducted by Harpending (Harpending 1976; Harpending and Wandsnider 1982) in 1967–8. Harpending obtained reproductive histories of about 500 !Kung women living in Ghanzi and throughout Ngamiland. Many of the !Kung living in Ghanzi were settled on cattle ranches and had been sedentary most of their lives. The !Kung ascertained by Harpending lived much the same way as those studied by Howell in the Dobe region. Harpending did not attempt to age !Kung, but because he distinguished between pre- and post-reproductive women and between infants and children, comparisons among all three data sets are possible.

Fertility

Popular explanations for low !Kung fertility

The quality of parental care

Low !Kung fertility has been attributed to wide birth spacing thought to be an adaptation to excessively high mortality among offspring whose births are spaced more closely than several years (Blurton Jones 1986) or because foraging women can only care for one small child at a time (Bleek 1928; Lee 1979). However, in a test of the Blurton Jones hypothesis and their own model of parental care, Pennington and Harpending (1988) found no relationship between offspring survival and the number of children a woman bears as predicted. Blurton Jones and Sibly (1978), Lee (1979), and Blurton Jones (1986) have emphasized increasing work loads of mothers with closely spaced births as fertility limiting factors.

Breast-feeding and the pace of child-bearing

Late age at weaning of children has also been suggested as a factor contributing to low fertility of !Kung women. Resumption of menstrual cycling post-partum is known to be delayed among lactating women. Prolonged breast-feeding leads to longer interbirth intervals, thereby reducing the number births a woman can fit into her reproductive span. Ovulation is thought to be inhibited most in mothers whose infants suckle frequently and intensely (Konner and Worthman 1980; Wood *et al.* 1985; Stern *et al.* 1986; McNeilly *et al.* 1988).

!Kung women breast-feed their babies on demand for several years contributing to substantial delays in the return of ovulation following parturition (Konner and Worthman 1980). Unfortunately, we do not have data on Herero with which to compare the contribution of breast-feeding to the spacing of their births. However, the Herero also breast-feed their babies on demand. They carry their babies tied to their backs throughout the day. The babies are removed and breast-fed whenever they cry or become restless. Both the Herero and !Kung introduce supplementary foods in the first few months of life.

Herero children are typically weaned in their second year of life. Many are then fostered either permanently or temporarily to relatives (see Chapter 8). No relationship between fostering and fertility was found among Herero. In contrast, the !Kung, who apparently do not foster their children, have been observed breast-feeding offspring as old as 4 years.

Extremely prolonged breast-feeding of women was thought to explain extremely wide birth spacing in !Kung women. Lack of suitable weaning food has also been suggested as the reason !Kung wean their children so late. These arguments hold to a certain degree, but because both the contraceptive effect of lactation and the proportion of calories that children obtain from their mothers' breasts decrease sharply during the second year post-partum, prolonged breast-feeding would not explain an average birth spacing of 4 years in a population. It is important to realize that pregnancy is a why reason !Kung wean their children, so that the effect of lactation on birth spacing cannot be measured from observational data alone. That is, prolonged breast-feeding may be an effect of sub-fecundity rather than a cause of it.

The possibility that !Kung reproductive function is impaired by thinness has also been raised (Howell 1979; Lee 1979; Bentley 1985). Low caloric intakes coupled with high energy outputs may cause !Kung women to ovulate irregularly or resume ovulation later post-partum. To what extent these mechanisms, if they exist, affect !Kung fecundity has not been measured.

Did more food lead to higher fertility?

Fertility of !Kung and Herero in the past

Age-specific fertility   A popular theme in anthropology and an integral part of the Bushmen legend is that sedentariness leads to higher fertility (Dumond 1975; Lee 1979; Handwerker 1983; Roth 1985). Campbell and Wood (1988), however, found that there was not a strong correlation between subsistence base and fertility levels. There is also little empirical support for this link for !Kung. Harpending and Wandsnider (1982) originally showed that contemporary populations of settled and nomadic women had identical levels of fertility, having an average of 4.03 and 4.08 births, respectively, at the end of child-bearing. Estimates from Howell's data of age-specific fertility from !Kung women who spent the majority of their reproductive years as nomadic foragers are slightly higher than for younger women, although many of the younger women were settled on ranches. Moreover, a comparison of !Kung and Herero fertility also shows that !Kung fertility is not unusually low when compared to other populations in this region and that sedentary populations, in fact, have lower fertility than !Kung.

Fig. 9.2 shows the age-specific fertility rates for Herero and !Kung calculated for the cohort of women who were post-reproductive in 1968 and for women reproducing in the period 1963–73. Age-specific fertility rates (ASFRs) are computed by dividing the number of live births to women in each age-class by the number of years at risk. The total fertility rate (TFR) is the sum of the age-specific fertility rates times 5 years (the width of the age-class). The cohort TFR is computed for women born in a defined period (women born before 1923 in this case) who have reached menopause. The Herero and !Kung cohort TFRs are based on births retrospectively reported by women. The period TFR is computed for all women who were of reproductive age at any time during 1963–73, regardless of when they were born. The !Kung period rates are based on observed births while the Herero rates are based on retrospective reports. The period TFR may be interpreted as the expected number of live births a woman would have at the end of child-bearing for a set of ASFRs. If fertility is constant through time, cohort and period TFRs will be equal.

The cohort TFR of Herero women who were post-reproductive in 1968 was only 2.7 compared to 4.7 among !Kung. In 1963–73, the Herero were characterized by a period TFR of 4.9, while the period TFR for !Kung was 4.3. The !Kung period rate reflects the experience of many women who had become relatively settled on Bantu (e.g. Herero) cattle ranches while the cohort rate reflects the experience of women who had spent most of their lives as nomadic hunter-gatherers. The plot of fertility rates (Fig. 9.2) and TFRs that summarize them, clearly show that fertility did not in-

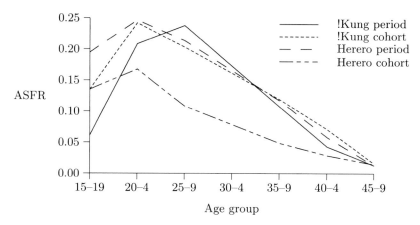

Fig. 9.2. !Kung and Herero period and cohort age-specific fertility rates (ASFRs). The cohort rates are from women post-reproductive in 1968. The period rates are from women reproducing in 1963–73. !Kung rates are from Howell (1979).

crease in response to sedentariness and the concomitant increase in food. Nomadic post-reproductive !Kung had higher fertility than sedentary post-reproductive Herero, and !Kung fertility did not increase in response to sedentariness. If anything, it appears that sedentariness caused lower fertility.

It is possible that the !Kung period rates are affected by age estimation errors as the age-specific fertility rates peak at an unusually late age. In natural fertility populations, the ASFRs typically peak among women aged 20–4 (Henry 1961; Wood 1989). Changes in infant mortality rates can also effect fertility rates. Women whose infants die before weaning may begin ovulating sooner so that declining mortality in a population can contribute to lower fertility rates. We show below that !Kung infant mortality rates have decreased. The difference is not large and would have very little influence on fertility rates. The difference in fertility rates between the sets of !Kung rates may be due to the lack of sterile women in the cohort of post-reproductive women (see below). In any case, it is clear that the !Kung did not experience a transition to higher fertility after settling on Bantu cattle ranches, although Herero fertility increased dramatically during this period.

It is also worth noting that the oldest !Kung women ascertained by Howell (1979, p. 125) had higher completed family sizes than those who had become post-reproductive more recently. Women aged 45–9, 50–4, 55–9, 60–4, and 65 or more had an average of 4.1, 4.2, 5.0, 5.0, and 5.3 births, respectively. This trend was confirmed in data recently collected by Patricia

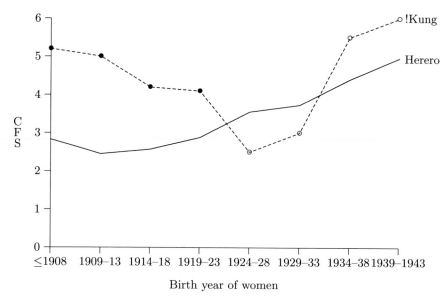

Fig. 9.3. Completed family sizes (CFSs) for cohorts of Herero and !Kung women since the turn of the century. !Kung data before 1924 (solid circles) are from Howell (1979). !Kung data after 1923 (open circles) are from Kranichfeld (1991).

Draper (Kranichfeld 1991). !Kung completed fertility apparently declined even further after Howell's research and, like the Herero's, is presently at its highest level since the turn of the century. We have plotted the CFSs of !Kung for 5-year birth cohorts in Fig. 9.3 using data published by Howell (1979) and Kranichfeld (1991). A plot of Herero CFSs is shown for comparison. We do not wish to make much of the differences between the Herero and !Kung rates indicated by the curves in Fig. 9.3. Most of the data points are calculated from small numbers of women so the error margins are wide.[1] Rather, we wish to emphasize the overall trends in the two curves.

The figure indicates that !Kung fertility was lowest among women born in 1924–8. This is the age group of women who were just beginning reproduction when the Herero migrated to the northern valleys around 1950. The apparent decline in fertility among !Kung born before 1924 is probably due to the more gradual increase in contact between !Kung and Bantu in the first part of the century.

That older !Kung women report higher fertility than younger !Kung women is also important for methodological reasons. Demographers more

---

[1] The tabulations necessary to statistically compare the !Kung CFSs were not published by Kranichfeld (1991) so we cannot present them here.

commonly observe that older women report fewer births than younger women and attribute this finding to factors such as poor memory recall in older women (see Chapter 5). The opposite pattern in !Kung indicates that this is not necessarily a problem inherent to all demographic surveys based on retrospective fertility reports. Most significantly, however, the downward trend in fertility clearly indicates that the low !Kung fertility was more recent than previously believed. !Kung fertility apparently declined by more than three births per woman in less than three decades.

Regional variation in Botswana   The reproductive rates of !Kung and Herero can also be compared to estimates based on the 1971 national census of Botswana, which included regional summaries of fertility rates (Central Statistics Office 1972). The TFR for Ngamiland in 1970 was 4.7, slightly lower than the period estimate of Herero. Only Orapa, Selebi-Pikwe, Ghanzi, and Gaborone had TFRs lower than Ngamiland. Orapa and Selebi-Pikwe are mining communities only recently settled at the time of the census. Ghanzi is a district bordering on the south of Ngamiland in which significant numbers of Europeans, Herero, and Bushmen (!Kung and other Khoisan-speaking groups) reside. The estimates of these three regions are based on small numbers. Gaborone is the capital of Botswana.

The average TFR in Botswana was 5.8. This estimate, computed from the raw data, was adjusted to 6.5 or more for various reasons (Central Statistics Office 1972; Finch and Way 1981). Adjusted figures by region were not given. Each of the three studies (of the Herero, !Kung, and population of Botswana) were conducted differently and subjected to different sources of bias. For example, the ages of Herero are certainly more accurate than the age estimates of !Kung and the population of Botswana. The !Kung estimates of period fertility are based on actual observations and are less likely to be biased by the reporting errors that can occur in retrospective studies, such as omission of births or confusion about the reference period. Both the Herero and !Kung figures are based on wide time periods and are less sensitive to annual stochastic fluctuations, although they are based on observations of fewer women. Regardless, all three studies estimate low levels of fertility in Ngamiland at the same time.

Estimates of past fertility reported in the 1971 census are also especially low in Ngamiland. For all of Botswana, women aged 45–9 reported having 5.6 births in their lifetime compared to an average of 5.2 births to women aged 50 or more. Except for Orapa, Ngamiland had the lowest averages in all of Botswana. Women aged 45–9 and 50 or more had only 4.0 and 3.8 births, respectively.

!Kung and Herero fertility transition in perspective   Although a thorough analysis of current !Kung fertility has not been published, a small study by Wilmsen (1986) reports that !Kung total fertility was 6.9 for the period 1976–80. Wilmsen argues that the increase is due to stabilization of the !Kung diet, but a similar if not more dramatic increase in fertility has been documented in the already-sedentary Herero (see Chapter 5). Herero period TFRs increased from a low of 2.7 in the first half of this century to 7.0 during the last decade. Wilmsen criticized a model of fertility proposed by Bongaarts (1982*b*) because it did not appear to fit Howell's estimates of !Kung fertility. Unfortunately, as Bongaarts pointed out in his rejoinder, Wilmsen failed to recognize the magnitude of primary and secondary sterility from sexually-transmitted diseases (STDs) in the !Kung. Bentley (1985) also discounted the contribution of STDs in her examination of the components of !Kung fertility when using Bongaarts' model.

Abnormally low rates of fertility are known throughout sub-Saharan Africa (see Chapter 6) comprising the well-known African infertility belt. As a secondary effect of anti-yaws campaigns in many parts of Africa involving widespread use of antibiotics (Guthe *et al.* 1972), the incidence of STDs declined, slowing the pace of infertility in those areas. In northern Botswana, the increase in fertility among Herero coincides with the introduction of mobile medical dispensaries. The pathologically low levels of fertility were apparently due to the sterilizing effects of pelvic infections in women, such as from the sequelae of gonorrhoea that can lead to pelvic inflammatory disease and blockage of the Fallopian tubes.

Because of the frequency of intermatings between !Kung and Bantu, it is likely that the !Kung also suffered from the devastating effects of STDs. Howell (1979) remarked upon the STD epidemic experience by !Kung following the movement of Bantu into the Dobe region in the 1950s. Even before Bantu moved into the northern valleys of Ngamiland, !Kung no doubt had opportunities for contracting STDs. Along the perimeters of their range in Angola, Botswana, and northern Namibia they have been in contact with peoples known to have a history of sub-fertility that we attributed to STDs in Chapter 6. The !Kung have a word for STDs in their own language ($\neq$ *unini*) indicating that it is not a new affliction. Interestingly, Howell dismissed STDs as being a complete explanation for low !Kung fertility. She estimated that STDs cost !Kung 3 per cent of their reproductive capacity per year during 1963–73 in comparison to the older women she studied. However, the older women also had low fertility, and fertility apparently declined throughout the early part of this century as the !Kung came into increasing contact with Bantu (Fig. 9.3). Since the older women were also probably afflicted by STDs, the total cost of STDs would be much higher.

In sum, low fertility was prevalent in Ngamiland at the same time that it was observed among !Kung. Adaptational explanations for changing !Kung fertility do not account for concomitant changes in fertility among other populations in the same region.

The length of birth intervals

One of the most convincing pieces of evidence for an association between sedentariness and transition to higher fertility was reported by Richard Lee who found that women he classified as 'more sedentary' had shorter interbirth intervals than women who were 'more nomadic' (Lee 1979, p. 322). However, there are several reasons to re-examine Lee's conclusions.

In his analysis, Lee estimated the mean number of months between live births to about 90 women who had at least two live births between 1963–73. The better nourished 'more sedentary' women had shorter interbirth intervals than the 'more nomadic' women. He also compared the mean number of months between births to women who had their two births in 1963–8 to women who had their two births in 1968–73. In both the nomadic and sedentary women there is a temporal decrease in the length of interbirth intervals which Lee believed reflected an increasing reliance on milk and cultivated grains in both groups. He emphasized differences in breast-feeding practices as an important factor.

In light of the Herero findings, Lee's conclusions are subject to an alternative interpretation. Because we know only the years in which Herero women had their births, we do not have comparable estimates of the length of interbirth intervals for Herero. However, since shorter birth intervals lead to higher fertility than longer birth intervals, we can compare trends in fertility between 1963 and 1973. Although differing levels of infant mortality can affect fertility levels, we show below that both !Kung and Herero had comparable levels of infant and child mortality during this period. Herero fertility increased steadily in 1963–73, and the temporal decrease in the length of !Kung birth intervals is probably due to the same factors that contributed to increases in Herero fertility. In addition to causing sterility, STDs contribute to fetal wastage and impede fecundity (see Chapter 6). Differences between more nomadic and more sedentary women may be due to the more sedentary women being better able to seek treatment for STDs because of their closer proximity to health posts as well as the medicines of anthropologists studying them. The presumably lower infection rates among Bantu in these areas also reduced the proportion of potentially infectious contacts at the cattleposts. Differences in breast-feeding practices may also be a factor.

The study by Lee also did not establish the causal direction of short birth intervals and sedentariness. He assumed that women became sedentary before their fertility increased when it is perhaps more plausible to assume that high fertility caused women to become sedentary. In other words, !Kung women who find themselves with closely spaced births have more incentive to become 'more sedentary' than women with fewer or more widely spaced births. This phenomenon was observed by Howell (1979, p. 50), who remarked, 'Families who are burdened with ...many children ...tended to congregate at the cattleposts in the 1960s, and the healthy members of the groups tended to gain weight on the high calorie diet available there'. Later (p. 210), in an analysis similar to Lee's, she noted that the most fecund women may be 'forced' to settle at the cattleposts because of their closely spaced births. This would result in a selective sample of the most fecund women being classified as 'less nomadic'. As we will show below, women with small children have the most to gain from settling as their children appear to survive better than the children of more traditional !Kung.

Lee's analysis can also be criticized on methodological grounds. First, he did not control for the effects of maternal age on birth spacing. The effect of age on fertility is obvious from Fig. 9.2, which shows that fertility declines steadily after peaking in the mid-20s. It is possible that Lee's results are biased by unequal age structures in the groups of women. Younger, more modern !Kung may find cattlepost life more attractive than older, more traditional women. Finally, Lee analysed only interbirth intervals that were completed during his study period. As Lee acknowledged, excluding censored birth intervals (intervals whose outcomes are still unknown at the conclusion of the study) can bias estimates of means since only short durations are included. This effect is obvious from the table presented by Lee in which the mean length of interbirth intervals that occurred throughout 1963–73 was substantially longer than those that began and finished in the two 5-year periods. Life table analyses are more appropriate for comparing sets of duration data since life tables can accommodate censoring (Kalbfleisch and Prentice 1980). It is possible, however, that Lee's results will be replicated by the more appropriate statistical analysis. Howell (1979) computed probabilities of closing birth intervals for different classes of women by weight and diet, but she did not establish that the groups of women had statistically different probabilities of having next births and did not consider the effects of age. It is feasible that the findings of Blurton Jones (1986), who found excessively high !Kung offspring mortality during short interbirth intervals and little or no mortality during long interbirth intervals, are similarly affected.

The estimates of completed family sizes from Harpending and Wandsnider (1982) also do not support Lee's interpretation. Harpending and Wandsnider describe two contemporary !Kung populations living under different subsistence regimes who had identical levels of fertility of four births per woman. Harpending and Wandsnider's estimates are based on reproductive histories of more than 200 post-reproductive women collected by Harpending (1976) at about the same time that Howell and Lee collected their data. The !Kung women classified as nomadic by Harpending lived throughout Ngamiland, including the Dobe region, and had spent their reproductive years as hunter-gatherers. The sedentary !Kung were women who had spent their reproductive years on Ghanzi cattle ranches. When the entire birth history of !Kung women is taken into account, there is no evidence that the lower activity levels and higher caloric intakes of sedentary women led to higher fertility.

The majority of the post-reproductive !Kung women ascertained by Harpending and Howell completed reproduction before antibiotics became widely available in rural Botswana. In contrast, Lee examined birth intervals of women who had differential access to health care during a period in which fertility was on the rise throughout north-western Botswana.

Harpending and Wandsnider's CFS estimates are somewhat lower than Nancy Howell's. This is probably due to Harpending's less precise definition of a live birth and the lack of sterile women in Howell's data. Harpending defined only children who lived long enough to receive a name (a few days) as live births. Although comparisons within the Harpending data can be made, some children die in the first few days of life so that the fertility of all !Kung women was slightly under-estimated. On the other hand, Howell probably over-estimated the CFS because she did not ascertain any sterile women. The primary sterility rate reported by Harpending and Wandsnider was about 10 per cent. If Howell's estimate is adjusted to accommodate this proportion of women with primary sterility, the agreement between the two data sets is quite good.

Howell speculated that the reason she failed to ascertain any sterile post-reproductive women was that sterile women selectively migrated to the cattle ranches (1979, p. 127). However, Harpending and Wandsnider (1982, p. 38) report that sterile women were ascertained in approximately equal proportions throughout Ngamiland. They suggested that sterile women were more mobile than women with children and were therefore classified as 'visitors' by Howell when she encountered them in the Dobe region. This also supports our interpretation that higher fertility causes women to become 'more sedentary' rather than Lee's interpretation that sedentariness causes higher fertility.

The length of the reproductive span

Age at first birth   Low fertility has also been attributed to late age at sexual maturity among marginally nourished women. Since the number of births a woman can have is affected by the number of years she has to reproduce, females who mature later may be able to fit fewer births into their reproductive spans. In contrast to the apparently lean !Kung of the 1960s, Herero are heavy and frequently suffer from obesity (O'Keefe *et al.* 1988) and are less likely to experience delayed sexual maturity due to nutritional stress. As pastoralists who maintain large herds of cattle and goats, they are relatively buffered against seasonal food shortages as well as drought. Therefore, if food affects fecundity (the biological ability to conceive) and the onset of sexual maturity, Herero women should begin reproduction earlier than !Kung. In addition, !Kung women living at cattleposts should reproduce at younger ages than foragers because they are heavier (Truswell and Hansen 1976; Howell 1979; Lee 1979).

It is standard practice to compute the mean age at first birth, but this is not a meaningful statistic for making comparisons between populations or between women who are at different points in their reproductive spans for several reasons. First, even women in natural fertility populations (populations in which birth control is not parity dependent) have first births at old ages. Comparing the mean age at first birth among women who are post-reproductive with those who are still reproducing can give the wrong impression that the age at sexual maturity has declined. This observation is often due to censoring women who eventually have a first birth but not until they are old. The mean is under-estimated because only women reproducing at the youngest ages are included in the statistic. In addition, not all women have first births, ever, and differences in primary sterility rates (the proportion of women who never have a live birth) between populations or cohorts of women can bias the estimate of the mean since the population at risk is ill defined.

The first problem can be avoided by computing the probabilities of having a first birth at each age and converting them into survivor curves. These are shown for the !Kung and Herero in Fig. 9.4. The curves are computed using the product-limit life table method (Kaplan and Meier 1958) described in Chapters 4 and 7 and given by the equation (Kalbfleisch and Prentice 1980)

$$\hat{F}(t) = \prod_{j \mid t_j < t} \frac{n_j - b_j}{n_j}$$

where $\hat{F}(t)$ is the survivor function, n_j is the number of women at risk of having a first birth at age j, and b_j is the number of first births occurring to women aged j. This yields the probability of not having a first birth by age t, conditional on the probability that a first birth has not already occurred. The product-limit life table method is similar to the more conventional actuarial method of estimating survivorship (usually denoted l_x in mortality studies) except that estimates are computed for every point at which an event (such as a birth or a death) occurs rather than for arbitrary intervals, such as 5-year age classes.

A comparison of the !Kung and Herero survivor curves for age at first birth for the cohorts of women who were post-reproductive in 1968 reveals that Herero women begin reproduction sooner, but that !Kung women 'catch up' and outpace Herero. As a whole, !Kung finish giving birth sooner

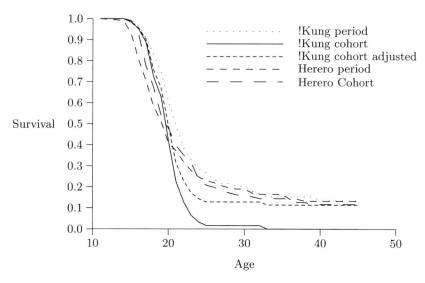

Fig. 9.4. Cohort and period survivor curves of age at first birth for !Kung and Herero. *Cohort* refers to women who were aged 45 or more in 1968. *Period* refers to women who were aged 15–44 at any time in 1963–73. The *adjusted* curve has 8 sterile women added. !Kung data are from Howell (1979).

than Herero, which is the opposite of what was expected. Log-rank scores provide statistics for testing the equality of survivor curves. The Mantel log-rank test in the SURVIVAL module of SYSTAT on an IBM PC compatible computer was used. The results are in Table 9.1. When survivor curves cross, log-rank statistics can give misleading results (Kalbfleisch and Prentice 1980). To mitigate this problem, we stratified the time axis at crossover points and computed X^2 statistics for sections of the curves (Kalbfleisch and Prentice 1980). Comparisons between the curves before and after the stratifications can be made. The degrees of freedom are equal to $r - 1$, where r is the number of curves being compared. A comparison of the two curves is made by summing the X^2 scores, with the degrees of freedom equal to $r - 1$ times the number of sections. The X^2 statistic for the section before the crossover is small, suggesting that the differences between the populations are due to chance. However, the statistic for the last portion of the curve is quite large, and the two scores summed together ($X^2 = 18.23$, 2 d.f.) suggest that the cohort of post-reproductive !Kung reproduce at a younger age than the Herero at a high significance level.

Much of the difference is due to the fact that there were no sterile women in Nancy Howell's group of post-reproductive women, a finding that is unusual even in populations with high levels of fertility. To make the

Table 9.1. Log-rank statistics for comparing equality of survivor curves. Cohort refers to women who were aged 45 or more in 1968, period refers to women who were aged 15–44 at any time in 1963–73. Scores for comparisons of Herero with !Kung cohort curves were stratified at the crossover points. !Kung data are from Howell(1979)

Comparison	Log-rank statistic	d.f.	p-value
Herero cohort vs !Kung cohort	1.39 + 16.84	2	0.00
Herero cohort vs !Kung cohort (adj.)	0.04 + .033	2	0.96
!Kung cohort (adj.) vs !Kung period	3.70	1	0.05
!Kung period vs Herero period	7.02	1	0.01
Herero cohort vs Herero period	0.09	1	0.77

populations more comparable, the !Kung curve was adjusted by assuming that the !Kung, like the Herero, had an 11.5 per cent primary sterility rate (equivalent to 8 sterile women). The results of applying the log-rank test to the adjusted data are given in Table 9.1. The statistic is small, indicating that the survivor curves for age at first birth in the two populations cannot be distinguished from each other.

Fig. 9.4 also shows the survivor curve for first births among women aged 15 through 44 in 1963–73. Some of the first births occurred before 1963. On the average, the !Kung cohort survivor curve reflects the experience of women who were older than !Kung women reproducing during 1963–73, after !Kung began settling among Bantu. Again, the effect is in the direction opposite to that expected. The period curve is higher than the cohort curve across all ages. The log-rank statistic using the adjusted data is 3.7 (1 d.f., $p = 0.05$). This means that women in 1963–73 had first births at older ages than the cohort of older, post-reproductive women.

Similarly, the comparison between the two period curves indicates that younger !Kung women also have a later age at first birth than younger Herero, and this difference is statistically significant. In contrast, the difference between the period and cohort curves for Herero is small and is statistically indistinguishable from zero. The log-rank statistic comparing the survivor curves is 0.090, 1 d.f., $p = 0.77$. Stratifying the time axis at the two crossover points results in a X^2 of 0.34, 3 d.f., $p = 0.95$.

Although the age at first birth of !Kung may have truly increased, the shift is more likely due to age estimation errors. We noted previously that the age-specific fertility rates during 1963–73 peaked at an unusually late age.

In sum, there is no evidence that the age at first birth, and therefore age of sexual maturity, of !Kung has decreased in response to more food or declining activity levels associated with sedentariness. Post-reproductive

!Kung women, who for the most part began their reproductive careers as nomadic foragers, began reproduction at the same ages as sedentary Herero. In addition, post-reproductive !Kung women began reproducing at *earlier* ages than !Kung reproducing in the period 1963–73. If anything, the evidence suggests that sedentariness caused an increase in the age at sexual maturity. No temporal change in the age at which Herero women begin giving birth was observed.

Age at last birth   Most of the difference in the level of fertility between the two populations is probably due to the average age at which women ceased child-bearing. Post-reproductive Herero women (in 1968) ceased reproducing at earlier ages, having their last births at 27 years of age, compared to 34 years for !Kung. The age at last birth for women who have completed reproduction more recently has increased. Seventy-four Herero women aged 45–54 in 1986 who had at least one live birth had their last birth on the average at age 32. Although there was no difference in the age at which these younger women began reproducing, the average number of births per woman (including 8 women who reported having no births) was 4.4. It appears that if Herero women continued to reproduce as long as !Kung, they would have about the same level of fertility.

The low fertility of Herero is attributable to women ceasing child-bearing early in their reproductive span (see Chapter 10). After considering a number of possible causes, we concluded in previous chapters that the sterilizing effect of pelvic infections in women is the best explanation for low Herero fertility in the early part of this century. The TFR for the period 1977–86 was estimated at 7.0 compared to 2.7 among the cohort of Herero post-reproductive in 1968. While there is no evidence that less work and more food affected !Kung fertility, the diminution of a single disease means that the average Herero women can expect to have four more births than she could only 30 years ago.

How food matters

In this section, the relationship between food and mortality is examined. Following Howell, mortality of !Kung offspring before and after about 1950 is compared. The year 1950 marks the acceleration of contact by !Kung with Bantu. The significance of more food for mortality is identified by comparing the magnitude of change in !Kung with Herero.

Pre-adult mortality

Herero and !Kung mortality estimated from reproductive histories during two periods indicates that mortality in both populations was higher in the past. Fig. 9.5 shows the survivorship, l_x, of the two groups for early and recent birth cohorts of children to age 15; l_x is the probability of surviving

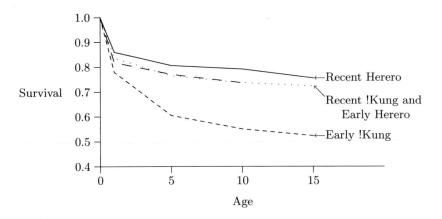

Fig. 9.5. Survivorship of !Kung and Herero offspring to age 15 before 1949 (early period) and 1949–68 (recent period). !Kung data are from Howell (1979).

to age x. The early !Kung period includes children born in the years 1919–48, and the early Herero period includes children born in 1917–48. The curves for the recent period are based on births occurring in 1949–68. Survivorship was computed for the first year of life (infancy) and for the age classes 1–4, 5–9, and 10–14. Howell observed no deaths in the age class of children aged 10–14 so l_{15} is not estimated.

The figure shows that Herero had lower mortality than !Kung in both periods but that recent !Kung mortality has declined to the low level of early Herero. Survivorship of !Kung children to age 10 in the recent period is 0.74 compared to only 0.55 in the early period. Although !Kung mortality decreased dramatically in the recent period, the drop in Herero mortality is substantially smaller, although the change is statistically significant.

The data from which the curves in Fig. 9.5 were calculated are given in Table 9.2. This table also gives the life table estimates l_x and 95 per cent confidence intervals. Quantity l_x is computed in the same way that the survivor curves for age at first birth were except that l_x is estimated only every 5 years since this is the form in which the !Kung data were published. The formula is

$$l_x = \prod_{j|x_j < x} \frac{n_j - d_j}{n_j}$$

n_j is the number at risk of dying during interval j, and d_j is the number of deaths to individuals in interval j.

Children who were not old enough to survive an age class were censored (i.e. information about them was discarded) at the beginning of the age interval, even if they died during the interval. The confidence intervals were

Table 9.2. !Kung and Herero offspring mortality to age 15 through 1968. Recent period is 1949–68. Early period is before 1949. !Kung data are from Howell (1979)

Population	Age-class	At risk	Deaths	l_x	Lower limit	Upper limit
Early Herero	0	293	48	1.00	1.00	1.00
	1–4	245	21	0.84	0.80	0.87
	5–9	224	8	0.76	0.71	0.81
	10–14	216	4	0.74	0.68	0.78
	15–19	—	—	0.72	—	—
Recent Herero	0	500	70	1.00	1.00	1.00
	1–4	303	19	0.86	0.83	0.89
	5–9	167	3	0.81	0.77	0.84
	10–14	66	3	0.79	0.74	0.85
	15–19	—	—	0.76	—	—
Early !Kung	0	258	57	1.00	1.00	1.00
	1–4	201	45	0.78	0.74	0.81
	5–9	156	14	0.60	0.55	0.66
	10–14	142	7	0.55	0.49	0.61
	15–19	—	—	0.52	—	—
Recent !Kung	0	231	42	1.00	1.00	1.00
	1–4	189	11	0.82	0.77	0.86
	5–9	68	3	0.77	0.71	0.82
	10–14	65	0	0.74	0.67	0.80
	15–19	—	—	—	—	—

estimated by applying the asymptotic normal distribution to a transformation of l_x as described by Kalbfleisch and Prentice (1980, pp. 14–15). The confidence intervals are given by

$$l_x^{\exp(\pm 1.96 s_x)}$$

s_x^2 is the asymptotic variance of $\log[-\log l_x]$ and can be estimated by

$$s_x^2 = \frac{\sum \frac{d_j}{n_j(n_j - d_j)}}{[\sum \log(\frac{n_j - d_j}{n_j})]^2}.$$

Log-rank tests are more concise statistics than confidence intervals for comparing survivor curves since they produce a single number rather than series of point estimates. Nevertheless, the confidence intervals still tell much of what we need to know. There is no overlap between the confidence intervals of the two early mortality periods, and the two !Kung curves overlap at only one point. Early Herero and recent !Kung are probably the same. Of the other two-way comparisons of interest (early Herero vs recent Herero and recent Herero vs recent !Kung), the overlap is at the extreme ends of the confidence intervals. Since the probability that all the true values of the point estimates fall at the extreme ends is less than 5 per cent, we can be reasonably certain that a decrease in mortality has occurred in both populations and that the Herero have lower mortality than !Kung.

Each Herero age class appears to have experienced increases in survivorship of roughly equal magnitude, with mortality being highest during infancy. In the early !Kung period, mortality during infancy and during the ages 1–4 were nearly equal. Interestingly, the large decline in !Kung mortality during the recent period occurred mostly among children aged 1–4. In this interval, the probability of dying declined from 0.22 to 0.06. This is nearly a fourfold decrease in mortality during the period of weaning and is probably due to the availability of milk.

The decline in !Kung mortality coincides with their settling among Bantu. Harpending and Wandsnider (1982) found a similar mortality differential between contemporary sedentary and nomadic !Kung. Infant mortality among the nomadic population was twice that of the sedentary group, and preadult mortality was about three times higher. The marked decrease in mortality among 1–4-year-old !Kung suggests that getting enough to eat is especially crucial during weaning. This may mean that nutritional stress is greatest among small children but does not imply an advantage to extremely wide birth spacing among foragers since the advantage is gained from domestic livestock. The proportion of calories that children receive from their mothers' breasts and the amount of breast-milk that women produce decline steeply after about 6 months post-partum (Harpending *et al.* 1990).

The mortality of Herero and !Kung during early life can be compared with estimates from the 1971 Botswana census. Finch and Way (1981) estimated the infant mortality rate for both sexes to be 97 per 1000 between 1964 and 1971. This compares with 140 per 1000 for Herero and 182 per thousand for !Kung during 1949–68. Estimates of l_{10} for males and females between 1964 and 1971 in Botswana were 0.81 and 0.84 (Finch and Way 1981; Central Statistics Office 1972) compared to 0.79 and 0.74 for Herero and !Kung for the sexes combined.

The higher estimates of mortality among !Kung and Herero are probably due primarily to higher overall levels of mortality in Ngamiland. Geographic breakdowns in survivorship reported by the 1971 census indicate that this region has the highest mortality in the country (Central Statistics Office 1972). Some variation may be due to differences in the methods

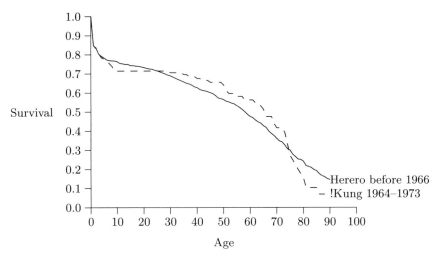

Fig. 9.6. !Kung and Herero survivorship throughout the life-span. The Herero curve is from Chapter 4. !Kung estimates are from Howell (1979). Both survivor curves correspond to life tables with an expectation of life at birth of 51 years.

used to calculate the estimates. The comparisons also reflect estimates of mortality for slightly different time periods. Some temporal decrease in mortality would be expected in the !Kung and Herero. We reported in Chapter 3 that Herero infant mortality in 1960–74 was only 120 per 1000.

The decrease in !Kung mortality means that the average child born after 1948 has about a 25 per cent greater chance of surviving to age 15, about the age of adulthood. (The empirical estimate of l_{15} during the recent period is the same as l_{10} but would be 0.72 if early Herero and recent !Kung mortality were the same.) This nets a considerable increase in the reproductive success of !Kung women. A 25 per cent increase in offspring survivorship is equivalent to a woman with four births increasing her reproductive rate by one more birth.

Mortality throughout the life-span

A comparison of Herero and !Kung survivorship throughout the life-span is shown in Fig. 9.6. The Herero survivor curve, taken from Chapter 4, is estimated from parents reporting the mortality of their children and children reporting the mortality of their parents. The curve shows the experience of Herero living in the period 1894 to 1965. The !Kung survivor curve is taken from Howell (1979) and is based on deaths observed in 1964–73. Both curves combine the experiences of both sexes and are remarkably similar.

The life expectancy at birth of a population can be used as a summary statistic for comparing populations. Both curves reflect life tables with life expectancies at birth of 51 years, further indicating that the Herero and recent !Kung are characterized by similar mortality schedules. Interestingly, Howell (1979) discounted her estimates of mortality, believing that !Kung mortality was much higher. At that time, however, she believed that the life expectancy at birth in Botswana was only 40 (Howell 1979, p. 95) so that the !Kung appeared to survive better than the general population. Estimates based on the 1971 Botswana census indicate that the population's life expectancy at birth during 1964–71 was 55 years (Finch and Way 1981). When contrasted with other estimates for Botswana, her estimates of !Kung survivorship are quite reasonable.

Summary

In this chapter we re-examined the demographic rates of !Kung Bushmen and evaluated the myth that the conditions of their foraging way of life were responsible for their fertility and mortality. We suggest instead that both were consequences of contact with Bantu pastoralists.

Fertility before and after transition to a more sedentary life-style among !Kung was compared and contrasted with the fertility of sedentary Herero. Although sedentary !Kung women had steadier food supplies and lower activity levels than nomadic !Kung, fertility did not increase after they began settling. In fact, older !Kung had higher fertility than !Kung women reproducing in 1963–73, although more than a decade had transpired since the !Kung started to become sedentary. Post-reproductive !Kung who had spent most of their reproductive span as nomadic foragers also had higher fertility than already-sedentary Herero. In addition, there were no differences in the ages at which Herero and post-reproductive !Kung women began child-bearing. The comparisons show that low fertility is a regional attribute and is not unique to marginally nourished foragers who get a lot of exercise. This conclusion is borne out by comparisons with the 1971 Botswana census in which Ngamiland had fertility rates that were among the lowest in the country. Previous explanations for low !Kung fertility are not general enough to account for low fertility throughout this region.

One might argue that !Kung sedentariness was too recent to affect reproductive performance. However, a comparison of their mortality before and after contact with Bantu indicates that !Kung were benefiting from sedentariness. Since the 1950s, when contact between !Kung and Bantu began increasing dramatically, survivorship of offspring to age 10 has increased by about 25 per cent. Most of the decrease in mortality occurred among children 1–4 years old, the age interval during which children are weaned. The mortality of these children declined by almost 75 per cent from a rate of 0.22–0.06.

The decrease in mortality is attributed to increases in the availability of food because a decline of similar magnitude was not found among the Herero. Survivorship to age 10 among Herero increased by only about 6 per cent. Compared to !Kung, decreases in mortality were roughly the same in all age classes. The huge decrease in mortality among !Kung children aged 1–4 suggests that more food is most important during weaning.

The level of survivorship of !Kung offspring in 1949–68 rose to the level of Herero in an earlier period. As a result, !Kung mortality was only slightly higher than Herero in the 1960s. Life expectancy at birth in both populations was 51 years.

Altogether, these findings indicate that more food can have a tremendous impact on reproductive success through its impact on survivorship. The chance that a !Kung child survives to reproductive age appears to have increased by more than 25 per cent as an apparent consequence of contact with sedentary peoples. There is no evidence that availability of food regulated !Kung fertility.

Our study emphasizes the need for a more rigorous comparative perspective in anthropology to understand better the significance of findings from restricted populations. We also suggest that evolutionary ecology would benefit from shifting some of its current focus on fertility to mortality.

10

History and population change

Historical changes in Herero mortality and fertility documented in previous chapters show that the health of this population has improved remarkably in the last century. In this chapter, we use these findings to address important issues in Herero history. We also discuss how improvements in survivorship and reproductive performance correspond to changes in population growth rates, social structure, and individual reproductive success.

Several volumes have been written about the Herero–German War of 1904–07 (Bley 1971; Drechsler 1980; Bridgeman 1981). Although it is clear that well over half the Herero were killed during the conflict, the true toll extracted by the war is unknown. Those who escaped to Botswana became the ancestors of most of the Herero in this study. In the first part of this chapter we reconstruct the age structure of the founding Herero population in Botswana to learn more about the demographic implications of the war. We estimate the sizes of the 1906 refugee and present-day Herero populations in Botswana by projecting an inferred age structure using fertility and mortality rates from previous chapters. Our analysis shows that the number who fled to Botswana has been significantly underestimated and that children suffered the highest mortality during the war years.

In the second part of this chapter, we discuss the relationship between changes in Herero demographic rates and changes in social structure. The 1986 population pyramid suggests that there is a wave of births about every 22 years. Since generation times in human populations are typically longer, and since the period of a wave in a population approaching stability is approximately one generation long, it appears that the low fertility prevailing during the early part of this century has reduced the generation time and, consequently, the mean age of child-bearing in this population. We estimate generation time using the eigenvalues of four Leslie matrices that encapsulate the transition from very low to very high fertility schedules in this population. There are several implications of reduced generation times for individual reproductive strategies. We also examine the relative importance of changes in mortality and fertility on population growth rates.

Estimating the number of Herero

It is wellknown that many Herero escaped the German genocide campaign in Namibia by fleeing to Botswana, but how many Herero were saved is unknown. In this section, we shed some light on this important event in the history of Herero and northern Botswana. We construct a series of Leslie matrices from estimates of Herero fertility and mortality and infer the 1906 refugee age structure from Herero population pyramids recorded in the 1950s. We project the inferred population pyramid using the Leslie matrices and arrive at estimates of the number of refugees that there must have been to produce the present-day Herero population in Botswana.

The population projection matrix

The age structure of a population pyramid reflects the balance of births and deaths occurring among its members. The number of individuals at each age depends on the number of individuals who were born in the past and their chances of surviving each age. The number of new-borns in a year is determined by the number of mature females and the rate at which they reproduce. This process can be modelled with a population projection matrix. The properties of the matrix, developed by P.H. Leslie in the 1940s (Leslie 1945, 1948), are well known. The basic form of the Leslie matrix for the female population is

$$
A = \begin{bmatrix}
F_1 & F_2 & F_3 & \cdots & F_j \\
P_1 & 0 & 0 & \cdots & 0 \\
0 & P_2 & 0 & \cdots & 0 \\
\vdots & \ddots & \ddots & \cdots & \vdots \\
0 & 0 & \cdots & P_{j-1} & 0
\end{bmatrix}
$$

The diagonal entries P_i, $i = 1, 2, 3, \ldots, j$, are the probabilities that females in age class i survive from time t to $t+1$. The F_i entries in the top row are the expected numbers of births to females in the ith age classes from time t to $t+1$. Following convention, we have used 5-year age and projection intervals so that individuals in age class $i = 1, 2, 3, \ldots, j$ are aged 0–4, 5–9, and so forth, and each projection t predicts the population 5 years in the future. In the projection below, we have computed estimates for $j = 19$ age classes.

For convenience, we have projected the female population only. Since the number of females in a population is roughly half the number of males, a good approximation is possible using a one-sex model. More complicated two-sex models have not produced consistently more accurate projections (Keyfitz 1985).

A population is projected by multiplying the $j \times j$ matrix A by a $j \times 1$

vector of population. Each $n_i(t)$ in the vector

$$n'(t) = (n_1(t), n_2(t), n_3(t), \ldots, n_j(t))$$

is the number of females in age class i at time t. Term $n'(t)$ is the transpose of the column vector $n(t)$. Given a schedule of P_i and F_i, future population is predicted by iterating the process $n(t+1) = An(t)$.

There are several ways of estimating P_i. Since the probability that an x-year-old survives 5 more years is $l(x+5)/l(x)$, we estimate the probability that individuals in age class i survive 5 more years from

$$P_i = \frac{l(x) + l(x+1) + l(x+2) + l(x+3) + l(x+4)}{l(x-5) + l(x-4) + l(x-3) + l(x-2) + l(x-1)},$$

where $x = 5i$. This formula is a weighted average of survival at each age over the interval. The formula given by Keyfitz (1968) in which $P_i = L_i/L_{i-1}$, where L_i is the total number of years lived by individuals in age-class i, is probably more familiar to most human demographers. Our estimate is more precise since we have tallied survival at each age of the interval.

In Chapter 4, we computed survivorship for two periods, before 1966 and in 1966–86. The corresponding schedules of P_i are given in Table 10.1. We will use both survival schedules in the projection of population.

The F_i are the fertilities of females in the interval i. They differ from age-specific fertility rates because they take into account the probability that some females will die and fail to reproduce during the projection interval. In addition, females reproduce at different rates as they age during t to $t+1$. Following Caswell (1989, eqn 2.22), we estimated the fertilities using the formula

$$F_i = l(2.5)\frac{m_i + P_i m_{i+1}}{2}.$$

This formula is equivalent to those found in more standard demographic sources such as Keyfitz (1985) . Term m_i is the number of girl births to females in age class i. It is estimated by multiplying the annual age-specific fertility rate of females in the ith age class by the fraction of births that are girls and the width of the age class. We assume that the fraction of girls is always 0.488, which is the actual proportion of all Herero births that were female. The term $l(2.5)$, which is the probability of surviving half the projection interval of the first age class, is empirically estimated from the equation $[l(2) + l(3)]/2$ to be 0.827 during the early period and 0.932 during the recent period.

We have computed F_i for four periods using the age-specific fertility rates given in the Chapter 5. They are listed in Table 10.1.

Table 10.1. Survival and fertility in the next 5 years by period. P_i is the probability that a female in age class i survives the projection interval and F_i is the expected number of female births to women in age class i during the projection interval

i	P_i −1965	1966–1986	F_i −1956	1957–1966	1967–1976	1977–1986
1	0.9163	0.9571	0.0000	0.0000	0.0000	0.0000
2	0.9704	0.9940	0.0000	0.0000	0.0000	0.0000
3	0.9674	0.9947	0.1286	0.1713	0.2176	0.2195
4	0.9726	0.9842	0.3023	0.3748	0.5386	0.5659
5	0.9702	0.9804	0.2822	0.3832	0.5785	0.6467
6	0.9707	0.9937	0.1562	0.2908	0.4624	0.5518
7	0.9641	0.9843	0.0879	0.1794	0.3340	0.4420
8	0.9654	0.9772	0.0689	0.1131	0.2068	0.2717
9	0.9603	0.9610	0.0265	0.0540	0.0923	0.0960
10	0.9504	0.9771	0.0000	0.0136	0.0155	0.0166
11	0.9393	0.9696	0.0000	0.0000	0.0000	0.0000
12	0.9216	0.9574	0.0000	0.0000	0.0000	0.0000
13	0.9042	0.9539	0.0000	0.0000	0.0000	0.0000
14	0.8876	0.8796	0.0000	0.0000	0.0000	0.0000
15	0.8211	0.8220	0.0000	0.0000	0.0000	0.0000
16	0.8350	0.7941	0.0000	0.0000	0.0000	0.0000
17	0.8024	0.6850	0.0000	0.0000	0.0000	0.0000
18	0.5283	0.6216	0.0000	0.0000	0.0000	0.0000
19	0.3708	0.3692	0.0000	0.0000	0.0000	0.0000

The age structure of the refugee population

If birth and death rates are constant, a population will eventually grow at a constant rate and approach a stable age distribution. As a result, the proportion of population at each age will become constant from year to year, whatever the initial distribution (Keyfitz 1968; Caswell 1989). Meanwhile, perturbations that cause unusual features will persist and provide clues about history.

The population pyramid in the right panel of Fig. 10.1 is the smoothed 1986 Herero population pyramid from Fig. 2.3. The pyramid reflects the 1986 Herero age–sex distribution and shows an apparent wave originating early in this century. We suggested that the wave resulted from excessive mortality among subadult Herero during the war years. The centre panel of Fig. 10.1 is a redrawing of a population pyramid constructed by Gordon Gibson, who censused several Herero homesteads in Ngamiland in 1953 (Gibson 1959). The pyramid shows the age structure of 240 males and females by 5-year birth cohorts. The distribution of individuals born in

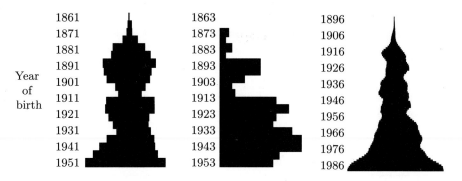

Fig. 10.1. Population pyramids of Herero in Botswana and Namibia. Left panel: the age–sex distribution of 7065 Herero in Namibia in 1951 compiled from four censuses. The left half of the pyramid shows the proportion of males, the right half shows the proportion of females. Centre panel: the age distribution of 240 male and female Herero in Ngamiland in 1953. Right panel: smoothed 1986 age–sex distribution of Herero in this study. Left side is males, right side is females. See text for sources.

1868–1903 in this pyramid reflects the distribution of population aged 0–40 in 1903, when the refugee Herero population was founded. A burst of births would follow as the population matured, and this birth surge would be echoed in subsequent generations. Although Gibson's sample is small, his pyramid is characterized by the same pinches and bulges suggested by our pyramid in the right panel of the figure.

Gibson's pyramid is also similar in shape to population pyramids from censuses of Herero conducted by Günther Wagner in Namibia in 1950–1 (Wagner 1957; Köhler 1959a, 1959b, 1959c, 1959d). A pyramid compiled from four censuses in these sources is shown in the left panel of Fig. 10.1. The pyramid reflects the proportions of population born in 5-year periods and reflects the age distribution of 3422 males and 3643 females. The censuses were taken on the Ovitoto (Wagner 1957), [1] Otjohorongo (Köhler 1959c), Otjiituuo (Köhler 1959b), and Waterberg (Köhler 1959d) Native Reserves. Although members of other tribes residing on these reservations may be included in the censuses, the reservations were occupied mostly by Herero. The largest census was of the Waterberg Reserve in which 1622 males and 1588 females were ascertained. At the Otjohorongo Reserve, Wagner censused 996 males and 1121 females. Both Waterberg and Otjohorongo were 95 per cent Herero in 1951. The Ovitoto and Otjiituuo

---

[1] The numbers of individuals in this census were reported for non-standard age classes. In compiling the numbers from the four censuses, we have assumed that the age classes 0–5, 6–10, 11–15,..., 96–100 used in the Ovitoto census corresponded to the age classes 0–4, 5–9, 10–14,..., 95–9.

censuses enumerated 111 and 693 males and 138 and 796 females, respectively. Over 80 per cent of the population in these reserves was Herero in 1951. None of the sources included details about how the data were collected.

Gibson (1959) attributed the pinch in 1904 to children dying crossing the desert to Botswana or because parents had to abandon them in Namibia. However, the same pinches are apparent in all the Herero pyramids of Namibia. It is more likely that the pinches are a result of an experience common to both populations, such as the war. They are not present in population pyramids of other ethnic groups in Namibia, such as the Tswana and Bergdama.

A deficit of young men and female children is apparent in the Namibian population pyramid. We do not know whether the asymmetry is due to differential mortality or to sex differences in migration patterns. For example, more young men than women may be away from the reserves because they have jobs in town, or the males may have died at a higher rate than their female age-mates. Wagner (1957) suggested that there were fewer girls than boys because girls were sent to live with relatives in urban areas (see Chapter 8) while boys were kept at home to help tend livestock. It is also possible that there were fewer female Herero children because they had higher mortality than males. We observed in Chapter 3 that, until recently, girls had higher mortality than boys. Although this finding is not statistically significant, the female deficit in the Namibian pyramid suggests that the differences in mortality may be real. Pennington and Harpending (1988) also observed a significantly higher mortality rate among the female infants of !Kung living at Ghanzi cattleposts in the 1960s but not among traditional !Kung hunter-gatherers. It is possible that female children were more susceptible than males to prevailing diseases, such as tuberculosis, at the cattleposts.

Despite its anomalies, the female age structure of the Namibian pyramid is a useful guide for inferring the population structure of Herero in Botswana after the war. We have approximated the 1906 female age distribution by structuring a pyramid that looks like the Namibian pyramids of 1951 after projecting it 45 years. The resulting inferred 1906 Herero population pyramid is shown in the left panel of Fig. 10.2. The centre panel, which compares the inferred 1906 pyramid projected to 1951 with the 1951 census data from Namibia, shows how well the inferred pyramid matches the actual data. The right panel compares the inferred 1906 pyramid projected to 1986 with the population pyramid from Fig. 2.2. Although the 1906 age structure was constructed independently of the 1986 population pyramid produced by our survey, there is congruence between the two pyramids.

We used the age distribution implied by the Namibian censuses rather

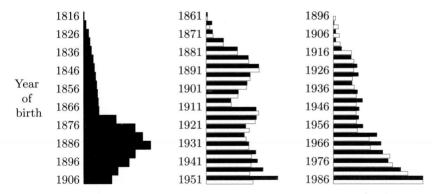

Fig. 10.2. Inferred and projected Herero population pyramids: 1906, 1951, and 1986. Left panel: inferred 1906 pyramid. Centre panel: the inferred 1906 pyramid projected to 1951 (hollow bars) is compared to the actual population structure of the 1951 Herero censuses in Namibia (solid bars). Right panel: the inferred 1906 pyramid projected to 1986 (hollow bars) is compared to the actual structure of the 1986 Herero pyramid constructed from this study (solid bars).

than Gibson's because the Namibian sample is much larger and is less likely to be biased by sampling error than the census of Gibson. Therefore, the Namibian data are probably more representative of the population structure of Herero in Botswana. Because most of the people older than 55 in 1906 (those born before 1866) were dead in 1951, we are unable to infer much about the 1906 age structure after this age. In drafting the 1906 pyramid in Fig. 10.2, we assumed that the proportion of Herero aged 45 or more declined at the rate predicted by the mortality estimates during the early period. It is possible that older people may have died at a higher rate than average because of wartime stresses. Age may have also rendered them less mobile and able to escape the Germans hunting them down. However, our approximation is a reasonable guess.

At the older ages, the inferred 1906 pyramid projected to 1951 matches the Namibian data well, but predicts too few children. The actual 1951 population of Namibia has 200 more females. We do not know to what extent the discrepancies are due to real differences in demographic rates and to what extent they are due to sampling error. It is possible that effective treatment for sexually-transmitted diseases (STDs) that cause sterility (see Chapter 6) became available in Namibia sooner than in Botswana, resulting in a higher birth-rate in Namibia in the 1940s. Even before antibiotics, Namibia had STD clinics on the reservations at which injections were administered (see Wagner 1957). A comparison of the Herero pyramids from the census by Gibson and from the censuses by Wagner in Fig. 10.1 supports this interpretation. The proportion of children in the Botswana population is much smaller than in the Namibian population. In any case, the close fit between the projected and actual 1986 Herero population suggests that the inferred pyramid is a good predictor of the 1986 population in Botswana and that there is a remarkable degree of consistency in our estimates of demographic rates. The increase in the birth-rate in the late 1950s is obvious.

The most remarkable feature of the inferred 1906 pyramid is the general deficit of population below the age of 20. Although it is possible that the pinch in the pyramid is due to pre-existing conditions, the tapering of population down to births occurring during the peak of hostilities suggests that it is due to excessive mortality among children during the war. The German genocide campaign caused the Herero to be unusually mobile. Most also lost all their livestock. Whether the excess mortality was due to sickness, starvation, or abandonment, children appear to have suffered the most during a period of conflict. The unusual age structure, present in both the male and female population, may have implications useful for studies of other historic and prehistoric populations. Deficits of subadults are not unusual in population pyramids constructed from prehistoric skeletal remains, although sample sizes are frequently too small and preservation of remains too irregular to draw firm conclusions about them.

Projection of the population

Although the number of Herero who came to Botswana in flight from the Herero–German War is unknown, previous research suggests that there must have been at least 2000 refugees. Tlou (1985) uncovered figures estimating that 500–1500 refugees settled in Botswana because of the war. Alnaes (1989) cites sources in which 200–300 refugees were counted in Ghanzi District and 1500 were counted in the Batawana Reserve (Ngamiland), so the number of refugees would be upwards of 1700–1800. A few hundred more Herero had already migrated to Botswana late in the nineteenth century. In 1946, when Botswana still enumerated its population by ethnic group, 5798 Herero were counted in Botswana (Research Publications 1973). The estimates of numbers of refugees and the 1946 enumerated population imply extraordinarily high annual growth rates of at least 2.8 per cent. The unusual age structure of the 1906 population would contribute to a more rapid increase than in a stable population, but the implied growth rate is probably under-estimated due to an undercount of population in the census. Although the quality of demographic data in Botswana has improved in recent decades, the 1946 government census was subject to large enumeration errors (Central Statistics Office 1981). The greatest difficulties occurred in remote areas like western Ngamiland, where even today there are few roads and population density is low. Given the low rates of fertility during the first half of this century, population growth of this magnitude is unlikely. As we will show below, the population in the first half of the century was nearly stationary.

Present-day estimates of Herero put their number at more than 10 000. Wilmsen (1982) estimated that there were 15 000 Herero living in remote areas of Botswana. Wilmsen did not state the year to which his estimate refers, but it is probably a rough estimate of their number in the late 1970s. Based on a survey of homesteads, Almagor (1982a) estimated that there were 5000 Mbanderu in the Lake Ngami area in 1978. Lake Ngami is the Mbanderu heartland, so Almagor's estimate included most Mbanderu in Botswana. Vivelo (personal communication, August 1990) guessed that there were 7000 Herero proper in Botswana in 1973. The two estimates combined indicate that there were about 12 000 Herero in Botswana in the mid-1970s. Although Vivelo was careful to distinguish between Herero proper and other Herero speakers in his estimate, his figure is based on communications that he had with government, medical, and veterinary officials of Botswana who may be less accustomed to making distinctions between the two groups. Many non-Herero we met in Botswana were not aware that Mbanderu are a separate people. We also knew many Herero proper and Mbanderu who had difficulty identifying themselves as only Herero proper or only Mbanderu. Herero proper and Mbanderu intermarry so many have relatives belonging to both tribes. Consequently, there is probably some overlap in the populations defined by Vivelo and Almagor as Herero proper or Mbanderu. Thus, 12 000 is probably an over-estimate of the number of Herero-speakers in Botswana. In our study, we ascertained about 3500 Herero-speakers living in Botswana in 1987–9. Since we sampled only a fraction of the total population, the number of Herero in Botswana today must be two to three times this figure.

To what extent the estimates of population at the various points in time agree can be assessed by projection. From the estimates of P_i and F_i in Table 10.1 above, we constructed four Leslie matrices describing population dynamics in the period through 1956 and in the periods 1957–66, 1967–76, and 1977–86. We then projected the inferred 1906 population age distribution to 1986. The sizes of the 1946, 1976, and 1986 Herero populations projected from a range of refugee population sizes are listed in Table 10.2.

From the table it is clear that the various estimates of population are not in accord. If there were only 2000 Herero in Botswana in 1906, the 1946 census enumerated several thousands more Herero than predicted by the population projection. If there were at least 6000 in 1946 and around 12 000 in the 1970s, then there must have been 6000–9000 Herero in 1906. These figures imply that there were 9400–14 100 Herero in 1986. Based on the frequency of multiple ascertainment of individuals in our study, our impression is that we sampled about one-quarter to one-third of the total population, suggesting that there were between 10 500 and 14 000 Herero in

Table 10.2.   Estimates of the number of Herero in Botswana in 1906–86. The 1946, 1976, and 1986 population sizes are predicted by projecting the inferred 1906 population pyramid from a range of starting values that represent hypothetical sizes of the refugee population. The last column shows how large the Herero population would have been had there been no infertility

| Number of refugees | Size of projected population | | | Without infertility |
1906	1946	1976	1986	1986
1000	1158	1292	1570	12371
2000	2315	2585	3139	24743
3000	3473	3877	4709	37114
4000	4630	5170	6279	49486
5000	5788	6462	7848	61857
6000	6945	7754	9417	74229
7000	8103	9047	10988	86600
8000	9261	10339	12557	98972
9000	10418	11632	14127	111343
10000	11576	12924	15696	123714

1986. A reasonable compromise of all these estimates suggests that there were about 8000 Herero in 1906 and that the population grew to about 12 500 in 1986. Since most of the 1906 population were refugees from Namibia, our analysis indicates that the number of Herero refugees has been significantly under-estimated. It appears that the people of Botswana saved many more Herero from the Germans than previously realized.

It is possible that migration of Herero into Botswana may bias these estimates. However, since Herero consider Namibia their homeland, most of the migration is in that direction. Therefore, if anything, there were even more refugees.

The last column of Table 10.2 shows how many Herero there would be had current levels of fertility prevailed throughout the century. If there had been no sub-fertility, the population of Herero in Botswana today would be 12 times its present size, regardless of its initial size. If our estimate of 8000 Herero in 1906 is correct, then there would have been nearly 100 000 in Botswana today. Instead of representing a very small fraction of the total population of Botswana, the Herero would have comprised about 10 per cent of all the people. Because the population of Botswana as a whole apparently did not experience pathological sub-fertility in the past, the Herero probably constitute a smaller fraction of the population today than they did after their flight from Namibia.

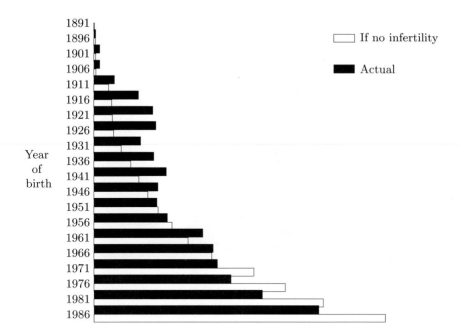

Fig. 10.3. Hypothetical age structure of Herero without sub-fertility. The hypothetical pyramid is contrasted with the actual age structure of the 1986 population constructed from this study.

Effect of sub-fertility on population age structure

Pathologically low fertility also appears to have resulted in a population structure in which the proportion of Herero grandparents to parents has shifted. Fig. 10.3 contrasts the actual 1986 population structure (from Fig. 2.2) with the age structure that would have resulted had the Herero reproduced at their current level of fertility since fleeing Namibia. This pyramid suggests that, for its current level of fertility, the proportion of grandparents to grandchildren is much higher than expected. The proportion of parents to children in the older generation is also higher than expected. The pinches and bulges apparent in the actual 1986 pyramid are not suggested by the hypothetical pyramid with the higher fertility rate.

The female side of the smoothed 1986 Herero age distribution from Fig. 2.3 reproduced in Fig. 10.4 also shows an apparent wave that we have already attributed to excessive mortality among subadults during the Herero–German War of 1904–07. Apart from its historical significance, the wave is interesting because it causes an unusual distribution of population. At every period of the wave, the number of children relative to the number

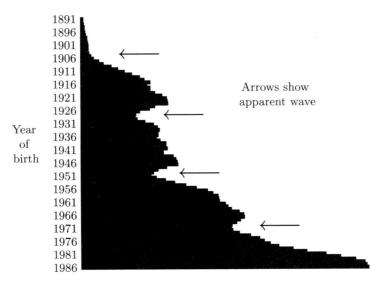

Fig. 10.4. Smoothed 1986 female population pyramid.

of adults fluctuates. This means that children born during the pinch have relatively more adult kinsmen to provide for them and that they will have fewer same-aged competitors than children born half a generation later. The pyramid also suggests that the length of the apparent wave is unusually short. Troughs in the apparent wave appear about every 22 years, several years shorter than calculations for most populations given in Keyfitz and Flieger (1971) . Since the length of a wave is generally longer in human populations, the short wavelength in the smoothed pyramid suggests that shortened reproductive spans resulting from STDs in the first half of the century may be responsible for increasing the frequency of oscillation in the pyramid and, consequently, for reducing generation time and the mean age of child-bearing in this population. We test this hypothesis and discuss its implications below.

Generation time and the length of waves

Natural periodicity is a characteristic of age-structured populations such that the wave resulting from a perturbation has a period about equal to the length of one generation (Keyfitz and Flieger 1971; Keyfitz 1972; Coale 1972). That is, given a fixed set of fertility and mortality rates, a surge of births occurring at a particular point in time will be echoed a generation later when the excess births mature to reproduce themselves. Thus, the length of the period $\mathcal{P}_2$ is approximately equal to the generation time T (Keyfitz 1968; Caswell 1989), where T is the number of years in which a population growing at a rate r will increase by a factor of the net reproduction rate (NRR), and the NRR is the expected number of baby girls born to a new-born female (e.g. Keyfitz and Flieger 1971).

Generation time can be derived from Lotka's renewal equation (Keyfitz and Flieger 1971) in which $e^{rT} = $ NRR so that $T = \ln(\text{NRR}/r)$. T has been shown to be equal to the mean age of child-bearing μ in the stationary population (Keyfitz 1968). In populations with positive growth, T is usually no more than 1 or 2 years less than μ (Keyfitz and Flieger 1971; Coale 1972). Since the length of the generation time reflects the age at which reproduction is concentrated, populations with longer generation times have reproduction concentrated at older ages compared to populations with shorter generation times (Coale 1972). The correlation between T and μ indicates that the average mother in populations with longer generation times will be older than in those with shorter generation times, and it follows then that, all things being equal, the average grandmother must be younger as well.

Generation time and population growth

The length of a population wave can be derived from its Leslie matrix. The eigenvalues of a Leslie matrix have their analogues in the Lotka integral equation such that $\ln \lambda_1 = r$, where λ_1 is the dominant eigenvalue of the matrix and r is the intrinsic population growth rate. For $i > 1$, the λ_i are complex so that their relationship to other roots r_i in the Lotka model are not one-to-one (Keyfitz 1968). Rather, the frequency of the natural periodicity is given by (Caswell 1989, eqn 4.38)

$$\mathcal{P}_2 = \frac{2\pi}{\tan^{-1} \frac{\Im(\lambda_2)}{\Re(\lambda_2)}},$$

where λ_2 is the second eigenvalue in magnitude with $\Im(\lambda_2)$ being the imaginary part and $\Re(\lambda_2)$ being the real part.

To test the hypothesis that infertility has reduced the frequency of oscillation in the Herero population, the series of Leslie matrices constructed for projecting the population were analysed to identify temporal changes associated with increases in fertility.

Results

The eigenvalues for each Leslie matrix were computed using routines in GAUSS by Aptech Systems on an IBM compatible PC. The annual growth rate $1/5 \times \lambda_1$ because we have 5-year projection intervals) and the second eigenvalue associated with the Leslie matrix for each period are listed in Table 10.3. The last column of the table lists the frequencies estimated using the formula for $\mathcal{P}_2$ above and multiplied by five, the length of the

Table 10.3. Population growth rates and the frequency of oscillation

Period	r	λ_2	$\mathcal{P}_2$
< 1957	−0.0051	$0.0852 \pm 0.7131i$	21.64
1957–1966	+0.0103	$0.1190 \pm 0.6830i$	22.47
1967–1976	+0.0309	$0.3640 \pm 0.6651i$	29.36
1977–1986	+0.0355	$0.3955 \pm 0.7223i$	29.37

age intervals. The λ_1 for the period of low fertility during the first half of the century indicates that, following their flight to Botswana, the Herero population was slowly declining at a rate of about −0.51 per cent per year. The intrinsic rate of population growth became positive following the recovery from infertility initiated in the mid-1950s. The population is currently growing at a rate of nearly 3.6 per cent per year.

The second eigenvalues show that the frequency of the natural periodicity in the population has increased from a low of 21.6 in the first period to 22.5 in the first 10-year period of recovery from infertility, to over 29 years in the last two decades. Comparisons with populations in Keyfitz and Flieger (1971) suggest that frequencies of less than 25 years are unusual. Of the populations studied, those with the shortest generation times tended to have low growth rates, but the pattern is not clear. Many populations with the highest growth rates had generation times of intermediate length.

Based on observations in teasel (a plant) populations in which a negative correlation between $\mathcal{P}_2$ and λ_1 was found, Caswell (1989) suggested that more rapidly growing populations may be associated with shorter generation times. Since increases in population growth rates among Herero are associated with longer periods of oscillation, Caswell's suggestion cannot always be true. Instead, this study suggests that the magnitude of the peak in reproductive rates may have the most dramatic effect on the frequency $\mathcal{P}_2$ in human populations. The curves of the age-specific fertility rates for the earliest periods (see Fig. 5.1) are relatively flat. The curve becomes sharply peaked following the period 1957–66, after which the most substantial increase in $\mathcal{P}_2$ occurs. While increases in fertility have resulted in dramatic increases in population growth rates, these increases are more gradual.

All else being equal, a short generation time means that women are younger, on the average, when they give birth. It also means that the grandmother of the average child in a population is also younger, and therefore more likely to be alive.

The intrinsic rate of population growth has increased dramatically among Herero in the last four decades. The rate of population growth across the continent of Africa as a whole is believed to have increased dramatically since the 1950s. Demographers have generally attributed these increases to declining mortality. This analysis of Herero, however, shows that decreases in sub-fertility had a much larger impact on population growth. Herero life expectancy at birth has increased by about 15 years. This big decline in mortality translates into only moderate increases in population growth rates. Substituting the P_i from the recent period into the diagonal of the two Leslie matrices for the periods before 1966 causes the population growth rates to increase to only -0.09 per cent and 1.5 per cent. Substituting the P_i from the early period into the two recent Leslie matrices causes the the population growth rates to increase to 2.7 per cent and 3.1 per cent. Although lower mortality has a significant impact on population growth, the effect is small in comparison to growth from increased fertility. The changes in mortality caused no changes in the estimates of generation time.

Dyson and Murphy (1985) also found that decreases in mortality cannot account for the increases in population growth rates observed in many developing countries. They attributed much of the increase in fertility to shorter birth spacing because of less breast-feeding but also to the reduction of sterility-causing diseases. Sub-fertility throughout Africa is well-documented, and the reduction of factors causing involuntary termination of child-bearing in women is surely responsible for large increases in the rate of population growth throughout Africa (Frank 1983).

Summary

A reconstruction and projection of the 1906 Herero population suggests that the number of Herero who came to Botswana as refugees of the Herero–German War of 1904–07 in Namibia has been significantly under-estimated. Based on the 1946 census, the projection indicates that there were at least 6000 refugees. Estimates of their number in the 1970s suggest that there may have been as many as 9000 refugees. These estimates imply that there are 11 000–14 000 Herero in Botswana today.

The shape of the present-day Herero population pyramid reflects the structure of its founding population, which was composed of a large proportion of females just entering their child-bearing years and a shortage of children. The ageing of these women into their peak reproductive years and a subsequent decline in the proportion of reproductive-aged women probably produced an apparent wave in the pyramid today. Evidence for infectious infertility afflicting this population through the mid-1950s can be seen in the narrow structure of the upper portion of the pyramid, while its recently broadened base is indicative of a gradual shift to higher rates of fertility. Because of their low levels of fertility, the Herero population has not increased much in this century. Our population projection suggests that there would have been between 75 000 and 111 000 Herero in Botswana today had their current level of fertility prevailed since their arrival as refugees. As a result, the proportion of population in Botswana represented by Herero has probably been declining.

The leading eigenvalue λ_1 of the Leslie matrix for the Herero population in the first half of this century indicates that population growth was -0.51 per cent per year. Recovery from infertility is responsible for transforming the Herero from a declining population into one experiencing extremely high population growth rates of about 3.6 per cent per year, a finding of great importance to policy planners in parts of Africa still characterized by high levels of involuntary infertility. The decrease in infertility has resulted in an increase in the period of oscillation in the population from about 22 to 29 years. Since the period of oscillation is approximately equal to generation time, which is correlated with the mean age of child-bearing in a population, these findings suggest that more children today are being born to mothers who are older than in previous decades.

We also examined the relative importance of declining mortality and increasing fertility on population growth rates. Although the decrease in Herero mortality contributed to increasing the rate of population growth, increases in fertility had a much greater impact.

References

Aborampah, O.-M. (1987). Plural marriage and fertility differentials: a study of the Yoruba of western Nigeria. *Human Organization*, **46**, 29–38.

Adadevoh, B. K. (ed.) (1974). *Sub-fertility and infertility in Africa*. Claxton Press, Ibadan, Nigeria.

Adepoju, A. (1978). Migration and fertility: a case study in south-west Nigeria. In *Marriage, fertility and parenthood in West Africa* (ed. C. Oppong, G. Adaba, M. Bekombo-Priso, and J. Mogey), pp. 491–506. Department of Demography, The Austrailian National University, Canberra.

Ahmed, J. (1986). Polygyny and fertility differentials among the Yoruba of western Nigeria. *Journal of Biosocial Science*, **18**, 63–73.

Allison, P. D. (1984). *Event history analysis; regression for longitudinal event data*. Sage Publications, Newbury Park, CA.

Almagor, U. (1980). Some notes on the Mbanderu calendar. *Botswana Notes and Records*, **12**, 67–82.

Almagor, U. (1982a). A note on the fertility of the Mbanderu women. *Botswana Notes and Records*, **14**, 23–25.

Almagor, U. (1982b). Pastoral identity and reluctance to change: the Mbanderu of Ngamiland. In *Land reform in the making: tradition, public policy and ideology in Botswana* (ed. R. P. Werbner), pp. 35–61. R. Collins, London.

Alnaes, K. (1989). Living with the past: the songs of the Herero in Botswana. *Africa*, **59**, 267–299.

Ambrose, S. H. (1982). Archaeology and linguistic reconstructions of history in East Africa. In *The archaeological and linguistic reconstruction of African history* (ed. C. Ehret and M. Posnansky), pp. 158–181. University of California Press, Berkeley.

Anderson, D. R., Sweeney, D. J., and Williams, T. A. (1981). *Introduction to statistics: an applications approach*. West, St. Paul.

Andersson, C. J. (1987). *Lake Ngami* (2nd ed.). C. Struik.

Armstrong, R. and Gilpin, M. (1977). Evolution in a time-varying environment. *Science*, **195**, 591–592.

Bean, L. and Mineau, G. (1986). The polygyny–fertility hypothesis: a re-evaluation. *Population Studies*, **40**, 67–81.

Begon, M. and Mortimer, M. (1986). *Population ecology: a unified study of animals and plants* (2nd ed.). Sinauer, Sunderland, MA.

Belsey, M. A. (1976). The epidemiology of infertility: a review with particular reference to sub-Saharan Africa. *Bulletin of the World Health Organization*, **54**, 319–341.

Bentley, G. (1985). Hunter-gatherer energetics and fertility: a reassessment of the !Kung San. *Human Ecology*, **13**, 79–109.

Betzig, L. L. (1988). Adoption by rank on Ifaluk. *American Anthropologist*, **90**,

111–119.

Blacker, J. (1984). Experiences in the use of special mortality questions in multi-purpose surveys: the single round approach. In *Data bases for mortality measurement*, pp. 79–89. United Nations, New York.

Blacker, J. and Brass, W. (1979). Experience of retrospective demographic enquiries to determine vital rates. In *The recall method in social surveys*, pp. 48–61. The London Institute of Education, London.

Bledsoe, C. and Isiugo-Abanihe, U. (1989). Strategies of child-fosterage among Mende grannies in Sierra Leone. In *Reproduction and social organization in sub-Saharan Africa* (ed. R. Lesthaeghe), pp. 442–474. University of California Press, Berkeley.

Bledsoe, C., Ewbank, D., and Isiugo-Abanihe, U. (1988). The effect of child fostering on feeding practices and access to health services in rural Sierra Leone. *Social Science and Medicine*, **27**, 627–636.

Bleek, D. (1928). *The Naron: a Bushman tribe of the central Kalahari*. Cambridge University Press, Cambridge.

Bley, H. (1971). *South-West Africa under German rule, 1894–1914*. Northwestern University Press, Evanston.

Blurton Jones, N. (1986). Bushman birth spacing: a test for optimal interbirth intervals. *Ethology and Sociobiology*, **7**, 91–105.

Blurton Jones, N. and Sibly, R. (1978). Testing adaptiveness of culturally determined behaviour: do Bushman women maximize their reproductive success by spacing births widely and foraging seldom? In *Human behaviour and adaptation* (ed. N. Blurton Jones and V. Reynolds), pp. 135–155. Taylor and Francis, London.

Bongaarts, J. (1981). The impact on fertility of traditional and changing child-spacing practices. In *Child-spacing in tropical Africa* (ed. H. Page and R. Lesthaeghe), pp. 111–129. Academic Press, London.

Bongaarts, J. (1982a). Does malnutrition affect fecundity? A summary of the evidence. *Science*, **208**, 564–569.

Bongaarts, J. (1982b). The fertility-inhibiting effects of the intermediate fertility variables. *Studies in Family Planning*, **13**, 179–189.

Bongaarts, J. and Potter, R. G. (1983). *Fertility, biology, and behavior: an analysis of the proximate determinants*. Academic Press, New York.

Bongaarts, J., Frank, O., and Lesthaeghe, R. (1984). The proximate determinants of fertility in sub-Saharan Africa. *Population and Development Review*, **10**, 511–537.

Boone, J. L. (1988). Parental investment, social subordination and population processes among the 15th and 16th century Portuguese nobility. In *Human reproductive behavior: a Darwinian perspective* (ed. L. Betzig, M. Borgerhoff Mulder, and P. Turke), ch. 12, pp. 201–220. Cambridge University Press, Cambridge.

Borgerhoff Mulder, M. (1989). Marital status and reproductive performance in Kipsigis women: re-evaluating the polygyny–fertility hypothesis. *Population Studies*, **43**, 285–304.

Boyd, R. and Richerson, P. (1985). *Culture and the evolutionary process*. University of Chicago Press, Chicago.

Brainard, J. (1986). Differential mortality in Turkana agriculturalists and pastoralists. *American Journal of Physical Anthropology*, **70**, 525–536.

Brass, W. (1958). The distribution of births in human populations. *Population Studies*, **12**, 51–72.

Brass, W. (1968). The use of existing data. In *The population of tropical Africa* (ed. J. Caldwell and C. Okonjo), pp. 172–178. Columbia University Press, New York.

Brass, W. (1975). *Methods for estimating fertility and mortality from limited and defective data*. International Program of Laboratories of Population Statistics, University of North Carolina, Chapel Hill.

Brass, W., Coale, A., Demeny, P., Heisel, D., Lorimer, F., Romaniuk, A., and van de Walle, E. (1968). *The demography of tropical Africa*. Princeton University Press, Princeton.

Bridgeman, J. (1981). *The revolt of the Hereros*. University of California Press, Berkeley.

Brittain, A. W. (1991). Can women remember how many children they have borne? Data from the East Caribbean. *Social Biology*, **38**, 219–232.

Brooks, A. (1989). Past subsistence and settlement patterns in the Dobe area: An archaeological perspective. Paper presented at the 88th Annual Meeting of the American Anthropological Association, Washington, DC.

Bullough, C. (1976). Infertility and bilharziasis of the female genital tract. *South African Medical Journal*, **83**, 819–822.

Caldwell, J. and Caldwell, P. (1983). The demographic evidence for the incidence and cause of abnormally low fertility in tropical Africa. *World Health Statistics Quarterly*, **36**, 2–34.

Caldwell, J. and Caldwell, P. (1987). The cultural context of high fertility in sub-Saharan Africa. *Population and Development Review*, **13**, 409–437.

Caldwell, J., Hill, A., and Hull, V. (1988). *Micro-approaches to demographic research*. Kegan Paul International, London.

Campbell, K. L. and Wood, J. W. (1988). Fertility in traditional societies: social and biological determinants. In *Natural human fertility* (ed. P. Diggory, M. Potts, and S. Teper), pp. 39–69. MacMillan Press, London.

Caselli, G. and Capocaccia, R. (1989). Age, period, cohort and early mortality: an analysis of adult mortality in Italy. *Population Studies*, **43**, 133–153.

Caswell, H. (1989). *Matrix population models*. Sinauer, Sunderland, MA.

Cates, W., Farley, T. M. M., and Rowe, P. J. (1987). Infections, pregnancies, and infertility: Perspectives on prevention. *Fertility and Sterility*, **47**, 964–968.

Cates, W., Aral, S. O., and Rolfs, R. T. (1988). Pathophysiology and epidemiology of sexually transmitted diseases in relation to pelvic inflammatory disease and infertility. International Union for the Scientific Study of Population, Johns Hopkins University.

Cavalli-Sforza, L. L. and Bodmer, W. F. (1971). *The genetics of human populations*. W. H. Freeman, San Francisco.

Central Statistics Office (1972). *Report on the population census 1971*. Gaborone,Botswana.

Central Statistics Office (1981). *Population and housing census. Census administrative/technical report and national statistical tables 1981.* Gaborone, Botswana.

Central Statistics Office (1987). *Population and housing census analytical report 1981.* Gaborone, Botswana.

Central Statistics Office (1988). *Statistical bulletin,* Vol. 13, No. 1. Gaborone, Botswana.

Charlesworth, B. (1980). *Evolution in age-structured populations.* Cambridge University Press, Cambridge.

Chojnacka, H. (1980). Polygyny and the rate of population growth. *Population Studies,* **34**, 91–107.

Clogg, C. C. and Eliason, S. R. (1987). Some common problems in log-linear analysis. *Sociological Methods and Research,* **16**, 8–44.

Coale, A. J. (1968). Estimates of fertility and mortality in tropical Africa. In *The population of tropical Africa* (ed. J. Caldwell and C. Okonjo), pp. 179–186. Columbia University Press, New York.

Coale, A. J. (1971). Age patterns of marriage. *Population Studies,* **25**, 192–214.

Coale, A. J. (1972). *The growth and structure of human populations, a mathematical investigation.* Princeton University Press, Princeton.

Coale, A. J. and Demeny, P. (1983). *Regional model life tables and stable populations.* Academic Press, New York.

Cohen, M. N. (1989). *Health and the rise of civilization.* Yale, New Haven.

Crawford, M. A. (1980). Lipid requirements during pregnancy and lactation. In *Nutrition and food science: present knowledge and utilization,* Vol. 3: *nutritional biochemistry and pathology* (ed. W. Santos, N. Lopes, J. J. Barbos, and D. Chaves), pp. 37–42. Plenum Press, New York.

Cronk, L. (1989). Low socioeconomic status and female-biased parental investment: the Mukogodo example. *American Anthropologist,* **91**, 414–429.

Cronk, L. (1991). Human behavioral ecology. *Annual Review of Anthropology,* **20**, 25–53.

Dawkins, R. (1976). *The selfish gene.* Oxford University Press, Oxford.

Deacon, H., Deacon, J., Brooker, M., and Wilson, M. (1978). The evidence for herding at Boomplaas Cave in the southern Cape. *South African Archaeological Bulletin,* **33**, 39–65.

Dickemann, M. (1979). Female infanticide, reproductive strategies, and social stratification: a preliminary model. In *Evolutionary biology and human social behavior* (ed. N. A. Chagnon and W. Irons), pp. 321–367. Duxbury, North Scituate, MA.

Doenges, C. E. and Newman, J. L. (1989). Impaired fertility in tropical Africa. *Geographical Review,* **79**, 99–111.

Dorjahn, V. R. (1958). Fertility, polygyny and their interrelations in Temne society. *American Anthropologist,* **60**, 838–860.

Dorjahn, V. R. (1959). The factor of polygyny in African demography. In *Continuity and change in African cultures* (ed. M. Herskovits and W. Bascom), pp. 87–112. University of Chicago Press, Chicago.

Draper, P. (1989). African marriage systems: perspectives from evolutionary ecology. *Ethology and Sociobiology*, **10**, 145–169.

Drechsler, H. (1980). *Let us die fighting*. Zed Press, London.

D'Souza, S. and Chen, L. (1980). Sex differentials in childhood mortality in rural Bangladesh. *Social Science and Medicine*, **6(2)**, 257–270.

Dumond, D. (1975). The limitation of human population: a natural history. *Science*, **187**, 713–721.

Dyson, T. and Murphy, M. (1985). The onset of fertility transition. *Population and Development Review*, **11**, 399–440.

Edlinger, M. (1988). Sexually transmitted diseases and fertility. A case study of Mahalapye Subdistrict, Botswana. Demographic reports No. 12, Geographical Institution, Groningen State University, The Netherlands.

Efron, B. (1977). Efficiency of Cox's likelihood function for censored data. *Journal of the American Statistical Association*, **72**, 557–565.

Efron, B. (1988). Logistic regression, survival analysis, and the Kaplan–Meier curve. *Journal of the American Statistical Association*, **83(402)**, 414–425.

Ehret, C. (1967). Cattle-keeping and milking in eastern and Southern African history: the linguistic evidence. *Journal of African History*, **8(1)**, 1–17.

Ehret, C. (1982*a*). The first spread of food production to Southern Africa. In *The archaeological and linguistic reconstruction of African history* (ed. C. Ehret and M. Posnansky), pp. 158–181. University of California Press, Berkeley.

Ehret, C. (1982*b*). Linguistic inferences about early Bantu history. In *The archaeological and linguistic reconstruction of African history* (ed. C. Ehret and M. Posnansky), pp. 57–77. University of California Press, Berkeley.

Ellison, P. T. (1990). Human ovarian function and reproductive ecology: new hypotheses. *American Anthropologist*, **92**, 933–952.

Fako, T. T. (1984). Historical processes and African health systems: the case of botswana. Ph.D. thesis. University of Wisconsin.

Farley, R. (1970). *The growth of the Black population*. Markham, Chicago.

Federick, J. and Adelstein, P. (1973). Influence of pregnancy spacing on the outcome of pregnancy. *British Medical Journal*, **4**, 753–756.

Fiawoo, D. (1978). Some patterns of foster care in Ghana. In *Marriage, fertility and parenthood in West Africa* (ed. C. Oppong, G. Adaba, M. Bekombo-Priso, and J. Mogey), pp. 273–288. Department of Demography, The Austrailian National University, Canberra.

Fienberg, S. E. (1980). *The analysis of cross classified categorical data* (2nd ed.). MIT Press, Cambridge.

Finch, G. S. and Way, P. O. (1981). *Country demographic profiles. Botswana*. US Department of Commerce, Bureau of the Census.

Frank, O. (1983). Infertility in sub-Saharan Africa: estimates and implications. *Population and Development Review*, **9**, 137–144.

Frank, O. (1987). The demand for fertility control in sub-Saharan Africa. *Studies in Family Planning*, **18**, 181–201.

Freed, R. S. and Freed, S. A. (1989). Beliefs and practices resulting in female deaths and fewer females and males in India. *Population and Environment*, **3**, 144–161.

Frisch, R. E. (1978). Population, food intake, and fertility. *Science*, **199**, 22–30.

Frisch, R. E. and McArthur, J. (1974). Menstrual cycles: fatness as a determinant of minimum weight for height necessary for the maintenance or onset. *Science*, **185**, 949–951.

Gage, T. B. (1989). Bio-mathematical approaches to the study of human mortality. *Yearbook of Physical Anthropology*, **32**, 185–214.

Gaulin, S. J. C. and Boster, J. S. (1990). Dowry as female competition. *American Anthropologist*, **92**, 994–1005.

Geldenhuys, P. J. and Hallet, A. F. (1967). Bilharzia survey in the eastern Caprivi, northern Bechuanaland and northern South West Africa. *South African Medical Journal*, **41**, 767–771.

Gelfand, M., Ross, M. D., Blair, D. M., and Weber, M. C. (1971). Distribution and extent of schistosomiasis in female pelvic organs with special reference to the genital tract. *American Journal of Tropical Medicine and Hygiene*, **20**, 846–849.

Gibson, G. D. (1952). The social organization of the Southwestern Bantu. Ph.D. thesis. University of Chicago.

Gibson, G. D. (1956). Double descent and its correlates among the Herero of Ngamiland. *American Anthropologist*, **58**, 109–139.

Gibson, G. D. (1959). Herero marriage. *Rhodes-Livingston Journal*, **24**, 1–37.

Gibson, G. D. (1962). Bridewealth and other forms of exchange among the Herero. In *Markets in Africa* (ed. P. Bohannan and G. Dalton), pp. 617–753. Northwestern University Press, Evanston.

Gibson, G. D. (1977). Himba epochs. *History in Africa*, **4**, 67–121.

Golbeck, A. L. (1981). A probability mixture model of completed parity. *Demography*, **18**, 645–658.

Goldman, N. and Pebley, A. (1989). The demography of polygyny in sub-Saharan Africa. In *Reproduction and social organization in sub-Saharan Africa* (ed. R. Lesthaeghe), pp. 212–237. University of California Press, Berkely.

Goodall, C. (1990). A survey of smoothing techniques. In *Modern methods of data analysis* (ed. J. Fox and J. S. Long), ch. 3, pp. 126–176. Sage Publications, Newbury Park, Calif.

Goody, E. (1973). *Contexts of kinship*. Cambridge University Press, Cambridge.

Goody, E. (1982). *Parenthood and social reproduction: fostering and occupational roles in West Africa*. Cambridge University Press, New York.

Goody, E. (1984). II. Parental strategies: calculation or sentiment?: fostering practices among West Africans. In *Interest and emotion: essays on the study of family and kinship* (ed. H. Medick and D. W. Sabean), pp. 266–277. Cambridge University Press, Cambridge.

Greenberg, J. (1963). *The languages of Africa*. Indiana University Press, Bloomington.

Gulliver, P. (1955). *The family herds; a study of two pastoral tribes in East Africa, the Jie and Turkana*. Routledge and Kegan Paul, London.

Guthe, T. (1962). Measure of treponematoses problem in the world. In *Proceedings of the world forum on syphilis and other treponematoses*, pp. 11–20. US Department of Health, Education, and Welfare, Atlanta.

Guthe, T., Ridet, J., Vorst, F., D'Costa, J., and Grab, B. (1972). Methods for the surveillance of endemic treponematoses and sero-immunological investigations of 'disappearing' disease. *Bulletin of the World Health Organization*, **46**, 1–14.

Hackett, C. (1953). Extent and nature of the yaws problem in Africa. In *First international symposium on yaws control* (monograph no. 15) (ed. WHO), pp. 129–182. World Health Organization, Geneva.

Hall, M. (1990). *Farmers, kings and traders; the people of Southern Africa 200–1860*. University of Chicago Press, Chicago.

Hamilton, W. D. (1964). The genetical evolution of social behavior, I. *Journal of Theoretical Biology*, **7**, 1–16.

Hamilton, W. D. (1966). The moulding of senescence by natural selection. *Journal of Theoretical Biology*, **12**, 12–45.

Handwerker, W. (1983). The first demographic transition: an analysis of subsistence choices and reproductive consequences. *American Anthropologist*, **85**, 5–27.

Harcourt, A., Harvey, P., Larson, S., and Short, R. (1981). Testis weight, body weight and breeding systm in primates. *Nature*, **293**, 55–57.

Harpending, H. (1976). Regional variation in !Kung populations. In *Kalahari hunter-gatherers* (ed. R. B. Lee and I. DeVore), pp. 152–165. Harvard University Press, Cambridge.

Harpending, H. and Chasko, W. (1976). Heterozygosity and population structure in Southern Africa. In *The measures of man* (ed. E. Giles and J. Friedlaender), ch. 9, pp. 214–229. Peabody Museum Press, Cambridge.

Harpending, H. and Draper, P. (1990). Estimating parity of parents: an application to the history of infertility among the !Kung of Southern Africa. *Human Biology*, **62**, 195–203.

Harpending, H. and Jenkins, T. (1973). Genetic distance among Southern African populations. In *Methods and theories of anthropological genetics* (ed. M. H. Crawford and P. L. Workman), pp. 177–200. University of New Mexico Press, Albuquerque, NM.

Harpending, H. and Pennington, R. (1990). Herero households. *Human Ecology*, **18(4)**, 417–439.

Harpending, H. and Rogers, A. (1990). Fitness in stratified societies. *Ethology and Sociobiology*, **11**, 497–509.

Harpending, H. and Wandsnider, L. (1982). Population structures of Ghanzi and Ngamiland !Kung. In *Current developments in anthropological genetics* (ed. M. Crawford and J. Mielke), pp. 29–50. Plenum Press, New York.

Harpending, H. and Ward, R. H. (1982). Chemical systematics and human populations. In *Biochemical aspects of evolutionary biology* (ed. M. Nitecki), pp. 213–256. University of Chicago Press, Chicago.

Harpending, H., Rogers, A., and Draper, P. (1987). Human sociobiology. *Yearbook of Physical Anthropology*, **30**, 127–150.

Harpending, H., Draper, P., and Pennington, R. (1990). Cultural evolution, parental care, and mortality. In *Health and disease in transitional societies* (ed. A. Swedlund and G. Armelagos), pp. 241–255. Bergin and Garvey, South Hadley, MA.

Heady, J. and Daly, C. (1955). Variation of mortality with mother's age and parity. *Lancet*, **February**, 395–397.

Henin, R. A. (1968). Fertility differentials in the Sudan (with reference to the nomadic and settled populations). *Population Studies*, **22**, 147–168.

Henry, L. (1961). Some data on natural fertility. *Eugenics Quarterly*, **8**, 81–91.

Hill, A. and Hill, K. (1988). Mortality in Africa: levels, trends, differentials and prospects. In *The state of African demography* (ed. E. van de Walle, P. O. Ohadike, and M. D. Sala-Diakanda). International Union for the Scientific Study of Population, Liège, Belgium.

Hill, A., Randall, S., and van den Eerenbeemt, M.-L. (1983). Infant and child mortality in rural Mali. Research Paper No. 83-5, Centre for Populations Studies, London.

Hill, K. and Hurtado, A. M. (1991). *Ache demography* (manuscript in preparation). Aldine, Chicago.

Hobcraft, J., McDonald, J., and Rutstein, S. (1983). Childspacing effects on infant and early child mortality. *Population Index*, **49**, 38–618.

Horn, H. S. and Rubenstein, D. I. (1984). Behavioural adaptations and life history. In *Behavioural ecology, an evolutionary approach* (2nd ed.) (ed. J. Krebs and N. Davies), pp. 279–298. Sinauer, Sunderland, MA.

Howell, N. (1976). Toward a uniformitarian theory of human paleodemography. In *The demographic evolution of human populations* (ed. R. H. Ward and K. M. Weiss), pp. 25–40. Academic Press, New York.

Howell, N. (1979). *Demography of the Dobe !Kung*. Academic Press, New York.

Huffman, S. L., Chowdhury, A. K. M. A., and Mosley, W. H. (1978). Postpartum amenorrhea: how is it affected by maternal nutritional status? *Science*, **200**, 1155–1157.

Hunter, G. W., Swartzwelder, J. C., and Clyde, D. F. (1976). *Tropical medicine* (5th ed.). W.B. Saunders, Philadelphia.

Huss-Ashmore, R. (1980). Fat and fertility: demographic implications of differential fat storage. *American Journal of Physical Anthropology*, **2**, 65–91.

Hytten, F. E. (1980). Nutritional aspects of human pregnancy. In *Maternal nutrition during pregnancy and lactation* (ed. H. Aebi and R. Whitehead), pp. 27–38. Hans Huber, Bern.

Ikels, C., Keith, J., and Fry, C. (1987). The use of qualitative methodologies in cross cultural research. In *Qualitative gerontology* (ed. G. D. Rowles and S. Reinharz). Springer, New York.

Irle, J. (1906). *Die Herero*. Bertelsmann, Gutersloh, Germany.

Isiugo-Abanihe, U. (1984). Prevalence and determinants of child fosterage in West Africa: relevance to demography. African Demography Working Paper No. 12, Population Studies Center, University of Pennsylvania.

Jacobson, L. and Weström, L. (1969). Objectivized diagnosis of acute pelvic inflammatory disease. *American Journal of Obstetrics and Gynecology*, **105**, 1088–1098.

Jenkins, T. (1972). Genetics polymorphisms of man in Southern Africa. Thesis, University of London.

Jenkins, T., Harpending, H., and Nurse, G. (1978). Genetic distance among certain Southern African populations. In *Evolutionary models and studies in human diversity* (ed. R. J. Meier, C. M. Otten, and F. Abdel-Hameed), pp. 227–243. Mouton, The Hague.

Johnston, F. E., Roche, A. F., Schell, L. M., and Wettenhall, H. N. B. (1975). Critical weight at menarche: critique of a hypothesis. *American Journal of Diseases of Children*, **129**, 19–23.

Kalbfleisch, J. D. and Prentice, R. L. (1980). *The statistical analysis of failure time data*. Wiley, New York.

Kaplan, E. and Meier, P. (1958). Nonparametric estimation from incomplete observations. *Journal of the American Statistical Association*, **53**, 457–481.

Keith, J., Fry, C., and Ikels, C. (1988). Community as context for successful aging. In *Cultural contexts of aging* (ed. J. Sokolovsky). Bergin and Garvey, South Hadley, MA.

Keyfitz, N. (1968). *Introduction to the mathematics of population*. Addison-Wesley, Reading, MA.

Keyfitz, N. (1972). Population waves. In *Population dynamics* (ed. T. Greville), pp. 1–38. Academic Press, New York.

Keyfitz, N. (1985). *Applied mathematical demography* (2nd ed.). Springer-Verlag, New York.

Keyfitz, N. and Flieger, W. (1968). *World population: an analysis of vital data*. University of Chicago Press, Chicago.

Keyfitz, N. and Flieger, W. (1971). *Population. Facts and methods of demography*. Freeman, San Francisco.

Kish, L. (1987). *Statistical design for research*. Wiley, New York.

Kitigawa, E. M. and Hauser, P. M. (1973). *Differential mortality in the United States: a study in socioeconomic epidemiology*. Harvard University Press, Cambridge.

Knodel, J. (1977). Breast-feeding and population growth. *Science*, **198**, 1111–1115.

Knodel, J. (1983). Natural fertility: age patterns, levels, and trends. In *Determinants of fertility in developing countries*, Vol. 1: *Supply and demand for children* (ed. R. A. Bulatao and R. D. Lee), pp. 61–102. Academic Press, New York.

Köhler, O. (1959a). *A study of Gobabis District (South West Africa)*, Ethnological Publications No. 42. Department of Bantu Administration and Development, Union of South Africa.

Köhler, O. (1959b). *A study of Grootfontein District (South West Africa)*, Ethnological Publications No. 45. Department of Bantu Administration and Development, Union of South Africa.

Köhler, O. (1959c). *A study of Omaruru District (South West Africa)*, Ethnological Publications No. 43. Department of Bantu Administration and Development, Union of South Africa.

Köhler, O. (1959d). *A study of Otjiwarango District (South West Africa)*, Ethnological Publications No. 44. Department of Bantu Administration and Development, Union of South Africa.

Kolata, G. (1974). !Kung hunter-gatherers: feminism, diet, and birth control. *Science*, **185**, 932–934.

Konner, M. and Worthman, C. (1980). Nursing frequency, gonadal function, and birth spacing among !Kung hunter-gatherers. *Science*, **207**, 788–791.

Kranichfeld, M. (1991). Cultural transition and reproduction among the Dobe area !Kung. Ph.D. thesis. The Pennsylvania State University.

Krebs, J. R. and Dawkins, R. (1984). Animal signals: mind-reading and manipulation. In *Behavioral ecology: an evolutionary approach* (ed. J. R. Krebs and N. B. Davies), pp. 380–402. Sinauer Associates, Sunderland, MA.

Kuczynski, R. (1949). *Demographic survey of the British Colonial Empire*, Vol. II. Oxford University Press, London.

Kurland, J. A. and Harpending, H. (1992). Sex dimorphism in growth and development of Herero: Differential parental investment? Submitted.

Lee, R. B. (1979). *The !Kung San*. Cambridge University Press, Cambridge.

Lee, R. B. and DeVore, I. (1976). *Kalahari hunter-gatherers*. Harvard University Press, Cambridge.

Leridon, H. (1977). *Human fertility: the basic components*. University of Chicago Press, Chicago.

Lesetedi, L. T., Mompati, G. D., Khulumani, P., Lesetedi, G. N., and Rutenberg, N. (1989). *Botswana family health survey II 1988*. Central Statistics Office, Gaborone, Botswana.

Leslie, P. (1945). On the use of matrices in certain population mathematics. *Biometrica*, **35**, 183–212.

Leslie, P. (1948). Some further notes on the use of matrices in population mathematics. *Biometrica*, **35**, 151–159.

Litschauer, J. and Kelly, W. (1981). *The structure of traditional agriculture in Botswana*. Division of Family Planning and Statistics, Gaborone, Botswana.

Lovejoy, C. O., Meindel, R., Pryzbeck, T., Barton, T., Heiple, K., and Kotting, D. (1977). Paleodemography of the Libben site, Ottawa County, Ohio. *Science*, **198**, 291–293.

Mabey, D. C. W., Ogbaselassie, G., Robertson, J. N., Heckels, J. E., and Ward, M. (1985). Tubal infertility in the Gambia: chlamydial and gonococcal serology in women with tubal occlusion compared with pregnant controls. *Bulletin of the World Health Organization*, **63**, 1107–1113.

Malan, J. (1974). The Herero-speaking peoples of Kaokoland. *Cimbebasia, Series B*, **2**, 113–129.

Mammo, A. and Morgan, S. P. (1986). Childlessness in rural Ethiopia. *Population and Development Review*, **12**, 533–546.

Manson-Bahr, P. H. (1950). *Manson's tropical diseases. A manual of the diseases of warm climates* (13th ed.). Williams & Wilkins, Baltimore.

Manton, K. G. and Stallard, E. (1984). *Recent trends in mortality analysis*. Academic Press, New York.

Manyeneng, W. G., Khulumani, P., Larson, M., and Way, A. (1985). *Botswana family health survey 1984*. Ministry of Health, Gaborone, Botswana.

Marshall, L. (1976). *The !Kung of Nyae Nyae*. Harvard University Press, Cambridge.

May, J. and McLellan, D. (1971). *The ecology of malnutrition in seven countries of Southern Africa and Portuguese Guinea*, Vol. 10, *Studies in Medical*

Geography. Hafner, New York.

McFalls, J. A. and McFalls, M. H. (1984). *Disease and fertility*. Academic Press, Orlando, Florida.

McNeilly, A. S., Howie, P. W., and Glasier, A. (1988). Lactation and the return of ovulation. In *Natural human fertility: social and biological determinants* (ed. P. Diggory, M. Potts, and S. Teper), pp. 102–117. MacMillan Press, London.

Medawar, P. B. (1957). *The uniqueness of the individual*. Methuen, London.

Medeiros, C. L. (1981). *Vakwandu: history, kinship and systems of production of an Herero people of South West Angola*. Junta de Investigações Científicas do Ultramar, Portugal.

Miller, B. (1981). *The endangered sex: neglect of female children in rural north India*. Cornell University Press, Ithaca.

Miller, B. (1984). Daughter neglect, women's work, and marriage: Pakistan and Bangladesh compared. *Medical Anthropology*, **8**, 109–126.

Ministry of Health (1982). *Medical statistics 1982*. Central Statistics Office, Gaborone, Botswana.

Mitchell, B. (1982). *International historical statistics: Africa and Asia*. New York University Press, New York.

Mooka, M. G. K. (1987). Introduction to Botswana society and culture. In *Population and housing census analytical report 1981*, ch. 1, pp. 1–7. Central Statistics Office, Gaborone, Botswana.

Morris, E. H. (1946). *Public health nursing in syphilis and gonorrhea*. W.B. Saunders, Philadelphia.

Muhuri, K. and Preston, S. (1991). Effects of family composition on mortality differentials by sex among children in Matlab, Bangladesh. *Population and Development Review*, **17**, 415–434.

Muir, D. G. and Belsey, M. A. (1980). Pelvic inflammatory disease and its consequences in the developing world. *American Journal of Obstetrics and Gynecology*, **138(7)**, 913–928.

Murdock, G. P. (1959). *Africa. Its peoples and their culture history*. McGraw-Hill, New York.

Musham, H. V. (1956). Fertility of polygynous marriages. *Population Studies*, **10**, 3–16.

Newell, C. (1988). *Methods and models in demography*. Guilford Press, New York.

Nortman, D. (1974). *Parental age as a factor in pregnancy outcome and child development*, Reports on Population/Family Planning, No. 16. Population Council, New York.

Nurse, G. and Jenkins, T. (1977). *Health and the hunter-gatherer*, Monographs in Human Genetics. S. Krager, New York.

Nurse, G., Tanaka, N., MacNab, G., and Jenkins, T. (1973). Non-venereal syphilis and Australia antigen among the G/Wi and G//Ana San of the Central Kalahari Reserve, Botswana. *The Central African Journal of Medicine*, **19**, 207–213.

Nurse, G., Harpending, H., and Jenkins, T. (1978). Biology and the history of Southern African populations. In *Evolutionary models and studies in human diversity* (ed. R. J. Meier, C. M. Otten, and F. Abdel-Hameed), pp. 245–254.

Mouton, The Hague.

Nurse, G., Weiner, J. S., and Jenkins, T. (1985). *The peoples of Southern Africa and their affinities*. Clarendon Press, Oxford.

Odahike, P. M. (1983). Evolving indications of mortality differentials by sex in Africa. In *Sex differentials in mortality* (ed. A. D. Lopez and L. Ruzicka), pp. 33–52. Australian National University Press, Canberra.

O'Keefe, S. J. D., Rund, J. E., Marot, N. R., Symmonds, K. L., and Berger, G. M. B. (1988). Nutritional status, dietary intake and disease patterns in rural Hereros, Kavangos and Bushmen in South West Africa/Namibia. *South African Medical Journal*, **73**, 643–648.

Oliver, R. and Fagan, B. (1975). *Africa in the Iron Age*. Cambridge University Press, Cambridge.

Oppong, C. (1989). *Growing up in Dagbon*. Ghana Publishing Corp., Tema.

Page, H. (1988). Fertility and family planning in sub-Saharan Africa. In *The state of African demography* (ed. E. van de Walle, P. O. Ohadike, and M. D. Sala-Diakanda), pp. 29–45. International Union for the Scientific Study of Population.

Page, H. (1989). Childrearing versus childbearing: coresidence of mother and child in sub-Saharan Africa. In *Reproduction and social organization in sub-Saharan Africa* (ed. R. Lesthaeghe), pp. 401–441. University of California Press, Berkeley.

Palloni, A. and Tienda, M. (1986). The effects of breastfeeding and pace of childbearing on mortality at early ages. *Demography*, **23**, 31–52.

Palloni, A., Massagli, M., and Marcotte, J. (1984). Estimating adult mortality with maternal orphanhood data: analysis of sensitivity of the techniques. *Population Studies*, **38**, 255–279.

Pebley, A. R. and DaVanzo, J. (1988). Maternal depletion and child survival in Guatemala and Malaysia. Paper Presented at the 1988 Annual Meetings of the Population Association of America, New Orleans.

Pebley, A. R. and Mbugua, W. (1989). Polygyny and fertility in sub-Saharan Africa. In *Reproduction and social organization in sub-Saharan Africa* (ed. R. Lesthaeghe), pp. 338–364. University of California Press, Berkeley.

Pebley, A. R. and Stupp, P. W. (1987). Reproductive patterns and child mortality in Guatemala. *Demography*, **24**, 43–60.

Pennington, R. and Harpending, H. (1988). Fitness and fertility in Kalahari !Kung. *American Journal of Physical Anthropology*, **77**, 303–319.

Peters, P. (1986). Household mangement in Botswana. In *Understanding Africa's rural households and farming systems* (ed. J. Moock). Westview Press, Boulder.

Phillips, R. (1989). Is early menopause a biological marker of health and aging? *American Journal of Public Health*, **79**, 709–714.

Phillipson, D. W. (1977). *The later prehistory of eastern and Southern Africa*. Heinemann, London.

Phillipson, D. W. (1985). *African archaeology*. Cambridge University Press, Cambridge.

Poewe, K. (1985). *The Namibian Herero. A history of their psychosocial disin-*

tegration and survival. Edwin Mellen, New York.

Research Publications (1973). *International population census publications, Botswana 1946.* Research Publications, New Haven, CT.

Richerson, P. and Boyd, R. (1989). The role of evolved predispositions in cultural evolution. *Ethology and Sociobiology,* **10**, 195–219.

Rogers, A. (1988). Does biology constrain culture? *American Anthropologist,* **90**, 819–831.

Rogers, A. (1990). The evolutionary economics of human reproduction. *Ethology and Sociobiology,* **11**, 479–495.

Rogers, A. and Harpending, H. (1986). Migration and genetic drift in human populations. *Evolution,* **40**, 1312–1327.

Rogers, A. and Harpending, H. (1992). Population growth makes waves in the distribution of pairwise genetic differences. *Molecular Biology and Evolution,* **9**, 552–569.

Romaniuk, A. (1968*a*). The demography of the Democratic Republic of the Congo. In *The demography of tropical Africa* (ed. W. Brass, A. Coale, P. Demeny, D. Heisel, F. Lorimer, A. Romaniuk, and E. van de Walle), pp. 241–341. Princeton University Press, Princeton.

Romaniuk, A. (1968*b*). Infertility in tropical Africa. In *The population of tropical Africa* (ed. J. Caldwell and C. Okonjo), pp. 214–224. Columbia University Press, New York.

Rosetta, L. and O'Quigley, J. (1990). Mortality among Serere children in Senegal. *American Journal of Human Biology,* **2**, 719–726.

Roth, E. (1985). A note on the demographic concomitants of sedentarism. *American Anthropologist,* **87**, 380–382.

Roughgarden, J. (1979). *Theory of population genetics and evolutionary ecology: an introduction.* Macmillan, New York.

Royston, E. and Lopez, A. D. (1987). On the assessment of maternal mortality. *World Health Statistics Quarterly,* **40**, 214–224.

Rushton, J. P. (1987). An evolutionary theory of health, longevity, and personality: sociobiology and r/k reproductive strategies. *Psychological Reports,* **60**, 539–549.

Sahlins, M. (1968). Notes on the original affluent society. In *Man the hunter* (ed. R. B. Lee and I. DeVore), pp. 85–89. Aldine, New York.

Salzano, F. M. (1971). Demographic and genetic interrelationships among the Cayapo Indians of Brazil. *Social Biology,* **18**, 148–157.

Schapera, I. (1945). *Notes on some Herero genealogies,* Communications from the School of African Studies, New Series No. 14. University of Capetown, Capetown.

Schapera, I. (1947). *Migrant labour and tribal life. A study of conditions in the Bechuanaland Protectorate.* Oxford University Press, London.

Serjeantson, S. (1975). Marriage patterns and fertility in three Papua New Guinean populations. *Human Biology,* **4**, 99–413.

Shaikh, K., Aziz, K., and Chowdhury, A. (1987). Differentials of fertility between polygynous and monogamous marriages in rural Bangladesh. *Journal of Biosocial Science,* **19**, 49–56.

Sieff, D. (1990). Explaining biased sex ratios in human populations: A critique of recent studies. *Current Anthropology*, **31**, 25–48.

Siegel, J. S. (1974). Estimates of coverage of the population by sex, race, and age in the 1970 census. *Demography*, **11**, 1–23.

Silk, J. B. (1987). Adoption and fosterage in human societies: adaptations or enigmas? *Cultural Anthropology*, **2**, 39–49.

Silk, J. B. (1990). Human adoption in evolutionary perspective. *Human Nature*, **1**, 25–52.

Silverman, B. W. (1986). *Density estimation for statistics and data analysis*. Chapman & Hall, London.

Simmons, G. B., Smucker, C., Bernstein, S., and Jensen, E. (1982). Post-neonatal mortality in rural India: Implications of an economic model. *Demography*, **19(3)**, 371–389.

Smith, J. E. and Kunz, P. R. (1976). Polygyny and fertility in nineteenth-century America. *Population Studies*, **30**, 465–480.

Solway, J. S. and Lee, R. B. (1990). Foragers, genuine or spurious? Situating the Kalahari San in history. *Current Anthropology*, **31**, 109–146.

Srinivasan, K. and Muthiah, A. (1987). Fertility estimation from retrospective surveys: biases attributable to pregnancy-related movement of mothers. *Demography*, **24**, 271–278.

Stearns, S. (1976). Life-history tactics: a review of the ideas. *The Quarterly Review of Biology*, **51**, 3–47.

Stearns, S. (1977). The evolution of life history traits: a critique of the theory and a review of the data. *Annual Review of Ecology and Systematics*, **8**, 145–171.

Stearns, S. and Crandall, R. (1981). Quantitative predictions of delayed maturity. *Evolution*, **35**, 455–463.

Steenkamp, W. P. (1944). *Is the South-West African Herero committing race suicide*. Unie-Volkspers, Capetown.

Stern, J. M., Konner, M., Herman, T. N., and Reichlin, S. (1986). Nursing behavior, prolactin and postpartum amenorrhoea during prolonged lactation in American and !Kung mothers. *Clinical Endocrinology*, **25**, 247–258.

Sudre, P., Serdula, M., Binkin, N., Staehling, N., and Kramer, M. (1990). Child fostering, health and nutritional status: the experience of Swaziland. *Ecology of Food and Nutrition*, **24**, 181–188.

Sundermeier, T. (1986). *The Mbanderu*. Michael Scott Oral Records Project, Windhoek, Namibia. Translated and edited version of *Die Mbanderu*, Collectanea Instituti Anthropos, Vol. 14, 1977.

Sween, J. and Clignet, R. (1978). Female matrimonial roles and fertility in Africa. In *Marriage, fertility and parenthood in West Africa* (ed. C. Oppong, G. Adaba, M. Bekombo-Priso, and J. Mogey), pp. 565–600. Department of Demography, The Austrailian National University, Canberra.

Symons, D. (1989). A critique of Darwinian anthropology. *Ethology and Sociobiology*, **10**, 131–144.

Timæus, I. (1986). An assessment of methods for estimating adult mortality from two sets of data on maternal orphanhood. *Demography*, **23**, 435–450.

Timæus, I. (1991). Estimation of mortality from orphanhood in adulthood. *De-*

mography, **28**, 213–227.

Tlou, T. (1985). *A history of Ngamiland–1750 to 1906: the formation of an African state*. Macmillan Botswana, Gaborone, Botswana.

Tolnay, S. E. (1989). A new look at the effect of venereal disease on Black fertility: the deep south in 1940. *Demography*, **26**, 679–690.

Trivers, R. L. and Willard, D. E. (1973). Natural selection of parental ability to vary the sex ratio of offspring. *Science*, **179**, 90–92.

Truswell, A. S. and Hansen, J. D. L. (1976). Medical research among the !Kung. In *Kalahari hunter-gatherers* (ed. R. B. Lee and I. DeVore), pp. 166–194. Harvard University Press, Cambridge.

Tumkaya, N. (1987). Mortality and life tables. In *Population and housing census analytical report 1981*, ch. 8. Central Statistics Office, Gaborone, Botswana.

Turke, P. W. (1989). Evolution and the demand for children. *Population and Development Review*, **15**, 61–90.

Ukaegbu, A. O. (1977). Fertility of women in polygynous unions in rural eastern Nigeria. *Journal of Marriage and the Family*, **39**, 397–404.

United Nations (1983). *Manual X. Indirect techniques of demographic estimation*. United Nations, New York.

van Dam, C. J. and Molosiwa, K. (1987). A control programme for sexually transmitted diseases in Botswana. Proposal to the Ministry of Health, Botswana.

van Warmelo, N. J. (1962). *Notes on the Kaokoveld (South West Africa) and its people*, Ethnological Publications No. 26. Department of Bantu Administration, Republic of South Africa. (Reissue of 1951 edition).

Vedder, H. (1966a). The Herero. In *Native tribes of Southwest Africa* (ed. C. Hahn, H. Vedder, and L. Fourie), pp. 153–211. Barnes & Noble, New York. Reprint of 1928 edition.

Vedder, H. (1966b). *South West Africa in early times* (trans. and ed. c.g. hall). Frank Cass & Co., London. Reprint of 1938 edition.

Vigilant, L., Stoneking, M., Harpending, H., Hawkes, K., and Wilson, A. (1991). African populations and the evolution of human mitochondrion DNA. *Science*, **253**, 1503–1507.

Vivelo, F. R. (1977). *The Herero of western Botswana: aspects of change in a group of Bantu-speaking cattle herders*. West, St. Paul.

Wagner, G. (1957). *A study of Okahandja District (South West Africa)*, Ethnological Publications No. 38. Department of Bantu Administration and Development, Union of South Africa. Revised and edited by O. Köhler.

Waldron, I. (1987). Patterns and causes of excess female mortality among children in developing countries. *World Health Statistics Quarterly*, **40(3)**, 194–210.

Wanless, J. F. (1938). Control of venereal disease. Unpublished MD Thesis.

Weiss, K. M. (1973). *Demographic models for anthropology*. Memoirs of the Society for American Archaeology, No. 27, Washington, DC.

Willcox, R. (1950). *A text-book of venereal diseases*. Grune & Stratton, New York.

Williams, G. (1957). Pleiotropy, natural selection, and the evolution of senescence. *Evolution*, **11**, 398–411.

Williams, G. (1966). *Adaptation and natural selection.* Princeton University Press, Princeton.

Wilmsen, E. (1982). Remote area dwellers in Botswana: an assessment of their current status. African Studies Center Working Paper, Boston University.

Wilmsen, E. (1986). Biological determinants of fecundity and fecundability: an application of Bongaarts' model to forager fertility. In *Culture and reproduction. An anthropological critique of demographic transition theory* (ed. W. P. Handwerker), pp. 59–89. Westview Press, Boulder.

Winikoff, B. (1983). The effects of birth spacing on child and maternal health. *Studies in Family Planning,* **14**, 231–245.

Winikoff, B. and Castle, M. A. (1988). The maternal depletion syndrome: clinical diagnosis or eco-demographic condition. *Biology and Society,* **5**, 163–170.

Wolf, M. (1972). *Women and family in rural Taiwan.* Stanford University Press, Palo Alto.

Wolfers, D. and Scrimshaw, S. (1975). Child survival and intervals between pregnancies in Guayaquil, Equador. *Population Studies,* **29**, 479–496.

Wood, J. W. (1989). Fecundity and natural fertility in humans. In *Oxford reviews in biology,* Vol. 11 (ed. S. R. Milligan). Oxford University Press, Oxford.

Wood, J. W. and Weinstein, M. (1988). A model of age-specific fecundability. *Population Studies,* **42**, 85–113.

Wood, J. W., Lai, D., Johnson, P. L., Campbell, K. L., and Maslar, I. A. (1985). Lactation and birth spacing in Highland New Guinea. *Journal of Biosocial Science Supplement,* **9**, 159–173.

Wood, J. W., Harpending, H., Milner, G. R., and Weiss, K. M. (1992). The osteological paradox: problems of inferring prehistoric health from skeletal samples. *Current Anthropology,* **33**, 343–370.

Wray, J. D. (1971). Population pressure on families: family size and child spacing. In *Rapid population growth* (ed. Nat. Acad. of Sci.), pp. 403–461. John Hopkins Press, Baltimore. Office of the Foreign Secretary, Washington, DC.

Wright, P. and Pirie, P. (1984). A false fertility transition: the case of American Blacks. Papers of the East-West Population Institute, No. 90. East–West Center, Honolulu.

Yerushalmy, J., Bierman, J. M., Kemp, D. H., Connor, A., and French, F. E. (1956). Longitudinal studies of pregnancy on the island of Kuaai, Territory of Hawaii. I. analysis of previous reproductive histories. *American Journal of Obstetrics and Gynecology,* **70**, 80–96.

Young, J. Z. (1971). *An introduction to the study of man.* Clarendon Press, Oxford.

Author Index

Subject Index

adoption 175
affluent society 97, 200
African infertility belt 16, 80, 103, 209
age exaggeration 47
age-heaping 47
age-ranking 47, 82, 203
age-specific fertility rates 103, 104,
    114, 205, 225
  !Kung 108, 205, 206
  Herero 52, 60, 103–8, 205, 206, 225,
    236
agriculturalists 18, 57, 72, 73
agriculture 38, 72, 102
amenorrhoea 128, 149
Angola
  !Kung 201, 209
  flooding of the Okavango 38
  Herero migrations 9–11
  Herero tribes 4, 6, 8
  Ovambo 8
  population density 16
  south-western Bantu 5
antbear 9
antibiotics 81, 108, 119, 135, 137, 209,
  212, 229
Arabs 81
ascertainment 76
asymmetric helping 65, 71

Baate 19
Baggara 115
Bantu
  contact with !Kung 108, 201, 205–7,
    209, 210, 215, 216, 219, 221
  Dobe region 19, 201, 202
  genetic relationships 12, 13
  Herero tribes 1
  Mozambique 14
  Namibia 14
  Ngamiland 4
  south-eastern 10, 11, 14, 16

south-western 5, 10, 11, 14, 16
Swazi 14
Western Highland 11
Bantu expansion 3, 5, 10, 11, 16, 34,
  136
Batawana Reserve 230
Bergdama 228
Bodibeng 37
Boers 6
Botswana
  Bechuanaland 5–8
  fertility 106, 107, 114, 115, 121–3,
    208, 209, 212
  inheritance 32
  mortality 1
    childhood 219
    infant 109, 219
    life expectancy 221
    sex differential 72
  offspring sex preferences 58, 64, 72
  per capita income 18
  persons per household 23
  STDs 103
Botswana Meat Commission 21
bride-wealth 64, 141, 142, 145, 165,
  181
British 6
Bushmen
  !Kung 1, 4, 12–15, 18, 19, 33, 41,
    47, 57, 70, 71, 75, 97, 103, 170,
    200–4, 208, 212, 222
    fertility 107, 108, 115, 121, 133,
      203–9, 213–6, 221
    health 125–7, 130, 209, 212
    infertility 16, 103
    mortality 57, 60, 75, 97, 210, 211,
      213, 216–22, 228
  G//ana 130
  G/wi 130
  Black 12
  Naron 13